Losing
the last
10 lb

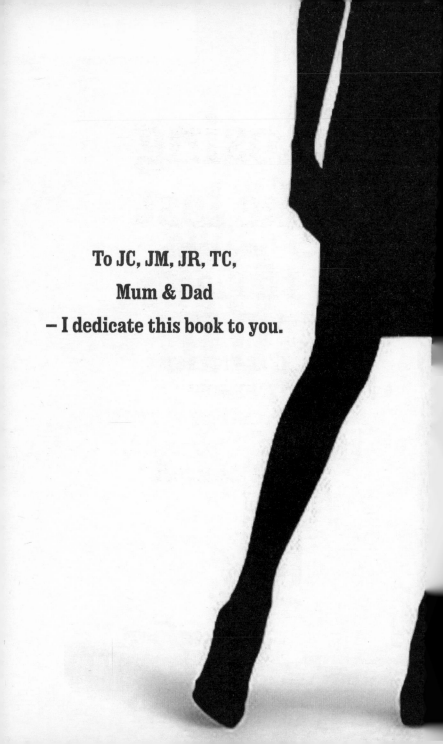

To JC, JM, JR, TC,

Mum & Dad

– I dedicate this book to you.

Losing the last 10lb

SIMPLE STEPS TO GET THE BODY YOU WANT NOW

susie burrell

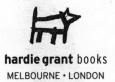

hardie grant books
MELBOURNE · LONDON

Contents

YOUR BEHAVIOUR

Check yourself

Sustainable change

YOUR BODY

YOUR LIFE

getting **STARTED**

'You've wasted enough time and energy on diets that get you nowhere. The time to get your food, your behaviour, your body and your life under control is now.'

Find your focus

'You are either committed to losing weight or you are not. There is nothing in between.'

One of the main reasons that many of us carry around extra weight is that it's so easy to gradually put on. It's easy to ignore, relatively easy to cover up and very easy to tell ourselves that such a small amount of extra weight doesn't really matter. We will lose it eventually.

To some extent we may be kidding ourselves, but when push comes to shove, if we set our minds to it, it's actually quite easy to lose the extra weight if we find and maintain our focus for a decent amount of time. Of course it would be nice to drop it in a few days, but when weight is lost that quickly it's generally water – not fat – and rarely achieved via sustainable methods. But if you're happy to spend just a few weeks minus your worst food habits and high-calorie treats, it's possible to lose – and keep off – your extra weight.

This book has been designed as both a quick-tip guide to dip into for those who already have a reasonably healthy lifestyle and just need a few tricks to get back on track, or as a full programme from start to finish for those who need to go right back to the drawing board. In my experience working with weight-loss clients for more than 10 years, it's not the super strict regimes that achieve sustainable weight loss long-term. It's the small but significant changes we can maintain for life that sees weight gradually shift for good. No matter what your starting point is as you grab this book, you will find useful tips and tricks that help you lose the weight for good.

Before you use this book as yet another weight-loss programme that you follow for a few days before becoming bored and reverting to your midmorning banana bread and caramel latte habit, can you commit the next 2–4 weeks to making a serious dent in your extra weight? Are you ready to prioritise your training so you don't skip your gym session, again? Are you ready to avoid your diet saboteur friends who offer you chocolates at work? Are you ready to rid yourself of your life-long diet mindset, which has taught you to believe that you have a slow metabolism and that you cannot lose weight? Are you ready to feel good?

While weight loss does not require you to be a diet and exercise purist, during the initial stages the more strict you are the better the immediate results will be. A small but significant weight loss experienced in the first few weeks of a new dietary regime is all you need to stay motivated and on track.

So, to move forward, clear your diary and get ready to commit to a good few weeks of healthy eating, exercise and taking control of your extra weight, once and for all.

Shift your mindset

'You have got to make conscious choices every day to shed the old – old issues, old guilt and old patterns.'

While most of us know how to eat well and stay healthy, it's often easier said than done. Busy lifestyles and family demands regularly result in health and fitness pursuits being put on the back burner, but it's our small, daily food and exercise choices that determine successful weight control. Fad diets, weight-loss challenges and boot camps may all have some short-term benefits for the mind and the body, but until health and fitness is viewed as a way of life as opposed to a short-term commitment, you are likely to find yourself back to where you started – signing up for yet another diet craze that takes you nowhere.

Once you prioritise looking after your body as part of your daily routine, the decisions that impact on your health are a whole lot easier to make. You don't even have to think about them. Instead of buying a pile of expensive, unappealing diet food on impulse to support a new fad regime, you automatically set aside time each week to buy the food your body needs to be at its best. You no longer have to deprive yourself of sweat treats because your desire to eat them has reduced. And most importantly, when you have indulged for a special occasion, you know what you need to do in order to get yourself back on track quickly.

Achieving the motivation and focus to implement such lifestyle changes develops gradually. First you need to admit that you are not feeling 100 per cent, and decide that you would look and feel much better if taking care of your body was part of your daily routine. Fuelling it with good-quality food, moving it regularly and keeping your intake of high-fat, highly processed foods to a minimum needs to become a habit, and the motivation to build and cement this habit has to come from somewhere deep within. Only this will drive you to do the things your body needs to be at its best, every single day.

To make changes to your health and fitness mindset, start by observing your current health-related behaviour. Take a look at your body in the mirror and see the evidence of where you have not been taking care of it. Think about how much better you would feel if you were fitter, or had less weight to carry each day. Then consider the easiest and most important changes you can make. Do you need to eat more vegetables and rely less on takeaway food? Are you choosing to drink water or sugar-laden soft drinks? Day to day, each food choice and exercise habit you reinforce contributes to your body shape and fitness level.

Why small changes work

'It's not the occasional burger or chocolate that ruins your diet – your daily routine controls your weight long-term.'

We have all tried them – ridiculously strict, exhausting diets that we stick to for a few days or even weeks before we eat something taboo and throw it all in. Introducing small dietary changes and regular exercise is a much more achievable alternative. While you will not see dramatic weight loss each week, unlike the various soup and shake programmes you have tried before, you will feel better instantly by losing and keeping off a small amount.

Too often we overcommit ourselves, becoming slaves to unreasonable goals and feeling disappointed and frustrated when we don't achieve them. We expect to lose weight in an instant, train for hours on top of long working hours and family commitments, have a buzzing social life, and prepare restaurant-style dinners and nutritionally balanced lunches for the following day. No wonder we fail – we set ourselves up for it.

Imagine if you could add one or two positive health changes to your day – snacking on vegetables or keeping your dinner small – and you could feel just as good and be losing weight at the same time. The good news is that you can. While allocating some energy and time to losing weight will help get you started on the right foot, the general rule is to only adopt changes that realistically fit into your life. Sustaining these small changes long-term will add up, and so too will your weight loss.

The power of planning

'Planning is the key to dietary success.'

It may surprise you to hear that it's planning, not knowledge, that is the key to dietary success. Most of us know what to eat, but in our busy lives, our healthy eating regimes fall off track when we find ourselves hungry and without any good food choices on hand. Sometimes we may be able to ignore the hunger pangs and wait until we stumble across an apple, but more commonly the deep desire for food sees us searching desk drawers or attacking vending machines for high-fat, high-sugar, carbohydrate-rich foods that feed our low blood sugar levels like a drug feeds an addict.

The simple act of planning ensures that we are never caught off guard. Ideally we should start each day knowing what we will eat for each meal and snack – what foods we need to take with us and what we are going to purchase. A simple rule of thumb is to always leave the house with a piece of fruit, two vegetables and some nuts. The fruit and nuts make a great midmorning or midafternoon snack, while the vegetables are always handy to munch on and ensure you are getting the daily bulk we need to feel full and satisfied.

Actively making time to get to the supermarket each week and stocking up on staples to prepare meals quickly is another key to success. Once a week, set aside half an hour to make a supermarket trip and stock up on nutritious, ready-to-eat snacks such as yoghurt, small tins of fruit, cereal and protein bars, long-life milk, breakfast cereal, low-fat crackers, packaged low-fat cheese and nuts. This range of food will keep you going for at least a week and ensure that you have an assortment of nutritious snacks to take with you to work, munch on before a workout or even make a quick dinner if you are too tired to cook.

If you detest supermarkets, maybe it's time to shop online. Convenient and time effective, online shopping not only means you are ready to eat well each week, but also means you avoid the temptation of buying extra foods you see when you find yourself at the supermarket hungry.

Power planning checklist

1 Shop once a week.

2 Know your quick, easy meals and keep a well-stocked pantry.

3 Have a big cook up once or twice a week to ensure you have leftovers for busier days.

4 Team up with a work colleague and start a lunch club. You provide two tasty lunches on Monday and Tuesday, they look after Wednesday and Thursday, then on Friday you can go out knowing you've had a healthy week.

5 Set aside 20 minutes on Sunday night to plan your meals for the week. This will make you less likely to fall into the takeaway trap.

6 Keep snacks with you at all times – each morning pack a couple of protein-rich snack foods to prevent impulse food purchases during the day.

7 Utilise lunchtimes. If you find it difficult to plan your food over the weekend, use lunch breaks at work to get to the supermarket.

8 Develop food rules. Create clear limits on when you will and will not eat certain types of food. For example, resolve only to eat out twice each week, this way you know when and in what context you will indulge, which will help with your diet goals.

9 Utilise helpers. There are many mums, partners and even friends who are often only too happy to help at home if you need it. Next time a member of your support team offers, ask if they will help you with a healthy meal or leftovers if you are finding it too difficult to fit meal preparation into your day. You might be surprised how happy they are to help.

Clean out the cupboards

'If you really don't want to eat it, throw it away.'

There are very few people who can keep highly appealing foods such as chocolate biscuits, potato crisps and other sweet treats at home without eating them. It's human nature to eat food when we see it. On top of the powerful visual stimulus food provides, we have the many years of food programming, courtesy of our parents, that teaches us from an early age about good and bad foods, and that we should limit the bad ones. This message of restriction quickly translates into wanting what we can't have and the inability to stop eating high-fat, treat foods when they are readily available to us.

A question I often ask my clients is, 'If I came and looked inside your cupboard, would I throw anything out?' In most cases, the answer is yes. The extra biscuits that are kept in case friends visit, the crisps that are for parties, the soft drink for the kids. These are foods few of us should be eating but we actively choose to keep such food in our visual field as a constant source of temptation.

Clearing out the fridge and the cupboards when you are about to commit to a new lifestyle regime is like a spring clean of your wardrobe. You cannot believe you kept those old daggy clothes around for so long and feel so much better once they're gone. The biscuits, chocolate bars, crisps, juice and soft drink all have to go. And before you say, 'But they're for the kids,' remember they are not good for the kids either. Once the cleanout is complete, replace the discarded items with key items you need on hand for those late nights returning home. Tuna, eggs, pasta sauce, pasta, low-fat cheese, frozen vegetables and potatoes can be converted into numerous quick, nutritious dinners in just 5–10 minutes.

Actively creating your own healthy environment, whether it's at home, your partner's place or at work, is absolutely crucial if you want to give yourself the best chance of staying on track with your new food regime. Remember, if tempting food is in front for you, you will want to eat it – you not weak or a glutton, you are simply human. Limiting your exposure to tempting treats is imperative as you strive to reach your diet and lifestyle goals, and it will make the process much easier!

DIET CORRUPTORS	CALORIES	CARBS (g)	FAT (g)
250g block milk chocolate	1300	155	70
100g cheese	360	0	32
50g potato crisps	260	24	16
1 chocolate biscuit	100	12	5
200ml fruit juice	80	18	0
10 plain rice crackers	70	15	2

Start with a detox

'Go hard or go home – true for life and true for weight loss.'

While the pros and cons of detox-style regimes are regularly debated in the media, the truth is they sell because if followed, they appear to work. To be honest, the physical effects aren't great – much of the weight lost is fluid as opposed to fat, and metabolic rate is compromised even after a few days of severe calorie restriction – but if the regime is specifically tailored to the individual by a health professional, and if the programme is followed for a short period of time only, the psychological effects of initial weight loss can be useful to keep individuals motivated to continue.

While there is no scientific evidence that the body needs to detox, or that a detox is effective in achieving sustainable weight loss, it offers an opportunity for you to refocus, establish clear goals, empowers you to concentrate on making healthy choices and, if done correctly, can see significant weight loss in a relatively short period of time.

Traditional diet programmes that eliminate 200–300 calories will at best result in a 1–2lb loss on the scales over a week. While that is the recommended rate of safe, lifestyle-friendly weight loss, psychologically this comparatively slow rate is often not enough to keep dieters on track. They feel their efforts have been in vain and search for other more rapid options. A couple of simple, short-term tricks, such as swapping breakfast for a shake or dinner for a soup, may give dieters enough of a drop on the scales to motivate them for longer.

Such programmes still include three meals and one to two snacks a day, but are lighter in total calories through particularly low-energy foods. Programmes like this need to be developed by a dietitian to ensure you don't reduce your calories to too great an extent and compromise your metabolic rate as a result. Following such a regime for just 3–5 days is likely to result in a drop on the scales, and if you reintroduce small amounts of energy-dense foods slowly, such as starchy vegetables, dairy and lean meat, you will continue to lose weight, although a little more slowly than during the detox regime.

The good news is that you don't need to fork out hundreds of pounds buying pills and potions to detox effectively. An effective detox can involve just cutting out the processed foods and stimulants, such as caffeine and alcohol, from your diet for a few days or a week to feel refreshed, re-energised and lighter, as your body rids itself of the excessive fluid it accumulates when too much salt and fatty food is eaten regularly.

To start your detox, stock up on plenty of fresh fruits and vegetables and base your main meals around them. Add some lean protein in the form of yoghurt, grilled fish, chicken or beans to your lunch and dinner, and drink plenty of water or herbal tea. Ditch the biscuits and processed bars for snacks – instead choosing fresh fruit or a handful of nuts and seeds. Wholegrain bread, oats and brown rice could also be included as sources of complex carbohydrates.

Generally speaking, any diet that contains fewer calories than you are used to leaves you vulnerable to hunger. A simple trick to avoid this, especially during the initial stages of a detox, is to eat a thick vegetable soup to provide bulk without many calories. A vegetable soup based on leek, celery, onions and garlic will not only provide nutrition but also help to draw excess fluid from the body, leaving you feeling light and less bloated. Try replacing both lunch and dinner with a vegetable soup for a couple of days at the beginning of your detox (see recipe on next page). As the soup consists entirely of vegetables, you can eat as much of it as you like for the remainder of the week – as a supplement to your lunch or dinner, or as a filling snack if you're hungry in between meals.

So if you are ready to drop the weight once and for all, now is the time to make a concerted effort to clear out your social diary and eliminate all extras from your diet for the first 2 weeks. Then you will be well on your way to sustainable weight loss.

DETOX SOUP

2 teaspoons olive oil

1 onion, finely chopped

1 leek, white part only, finely sliced and washed

1/2 head of celery, chopped

2 cups (500ml) salt-reduced vegetable stock

3 cups (750ml) water

400g tin chopped tomatoes

1 carrot, cut into 1cm cubes

500g pumpkin, peeled and cut into 1cm cubes

1 head of broccoli, cut into florets and steamed

1 Gently heat the oil in a large saucepan. Add the onion, leek and celery and sauté over a low heat until soft, for about 5 minutes.

2 Add the stock, water, tomatoes, carrot and pumpkin. Bring to the boil, then reduce the heat and simmer for 10 minutes.

3 Top with the steamed broccoli and serve.

Serves 6–8

Top 10 tips for a successful detox

1   Eliminate all alcohol and caffeine, including tea, coffee and cola drinks.
2   Eliminate all processed snack foods, such as biscuits, bars, cakes and cereals.
3   Eat at least 3 cups of vegetables or salad and 2 pieces of fruit each day.
4   Snack on fresh fruit or a handful of nuts.
5   Stick to lean proteins, such as chicken breast with vegetables/salad for main meals.
6   Include at least 1 cup of wholegrain carbohydrates each day for energy. Good choices include oats, beans, chickpeas and sweet potato.
7   Expect to feel tired and headachy for the first couple of days before feeling revitalised by day three.
8   Aim to drink 2–3 litres of water each day. More than this is not necessarily better.
9   Don't over-train during your detox – a 30–60 minute walk each day is more than adequate when you are not eating many calories.
10 Commit to a detox period of just 5–7 days.

	BREAKFAST	MID MORNING	LUNCH	MID AFTERNOON	DINNER
SAMPLE WEEKLY DETOX PLAN					
MONDAY	Glass of tomato juice + large bowl of fruit salad	Piece of fruit	Detox soup	10 walnuts + piece of fresh fruit	Detox soup + 100g tuna steak + steamed vegetables
TUESDAY	Glass of tomato juice + 200g natural yoghurt + fresh berries	Piece of fruit	Detox soup	10 walnuts + piece of fresh fruit	Detox soup + 100g salmon + steamed broccoli or pak choi
WEDNESDAY	Glass of tomato juice + ⅓ cup oats or muesli + 1 cup low-fat milk	Piece of fruit	1 cup brown rice + 100g tuna + sweet chilli sauce	10 walnuts + piece of fresh fruit	Detox soup + 100g grilled fish or chicken breast + mixed vegetables
THURSDAY	Glass of tomato juice + ⅓ cup oats + 1 cup low-fat milk	Piece of fruit	Mixed salad + 100g salmon + olive oil dressing + 2 slices of wholegrain bread	10 walnuts + piece of fresh fruit	Detox soup + prawn and vegetable stir-fry + ½ cup brown rice
FRIDAY	Glass of tomato juice + ⅓ cup oats + 1 cup low-fat milk	Piece of fruit	Turkey and avocado wrap	10 walnuts + piece of fresh fruit	Grilled Mediterranean vegetables + 100g chicken breast
SATURDAY	2 poached eggs + smoked salmon + 1 slice sourdough toast	Piece of fruit	Chicken breast wrap	OFF	OFF
SUNDAY	OFF	OFF	Omelette + low-fat latte	OFF	Detox soup

your **FOOD**

'*Your body is a temple that deserves to be nourished with good food.*'

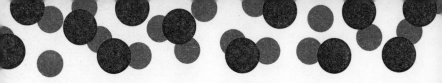

Eat more vegetables

'Just one piece of advice for better health and weight control – eat more vegetables.'

Of all the scientific evidence that points to keeping healthy and our body weight in check, eating plenty of vegetables wins hands down. It is also safe to say that the majority of us know that vegetables are good for us, so why do we not eat more of them?

When things get busy, for a number of reasons, it is the vegetable component of our evening meal that falls by the wayside. Meals purchased on the run or that are prepared quickly at home are often light on fresh vegetables – the downside of which is that we fail to get all the fibre, vitamins, minerals and bulk in the diet that we need to feel full and satisfied, leaving us prone to overeating.

Ideally an adult requires at least 3 cups of vegetables or salad every day, and the brighter the colour of the vegetables, the better they will be for you. Unlike fruit, which is carbohydrate-based, vegetables consist mainly of water so have virtually no calories, which means you can eat as many as you like without fear of weight gain. Eating plenty of nutrient-rich vegetables daily also means that you simply have less room in your diet for poor-quality food.

Diets rich in brightly coloured, fresh vegetables also have enormous benefits for cell health. Vegetables contain a complex array of phytochemicals, antioxidants and minerals that work in unison to protect cells from the damage linked to ageing, macular degeneration and even some types of cancer. While there are literally hundreds of supplementary forms of these nutrients, the evidence to date suggests that the health benefits are strongest when the real food forms are eaten.

In order to get enough vegetables in your daily diet, you need to have portions at both lunch and dinner. Order or make your sandwiches with lots of salad, or take an extra couple of salad vegetables with you to eat with your lunch. Juicing vegetables including carrots, celery and beetroot is another great way to incorporate them into your diet. Try enjoying them in soup for a lunch option or even raw as a pre-dinner snack. Dinner plates should be routinely half-filled with vegetables or salad. Make a concerted effort to always order extra sides of vegetables or salad when eating out.

By simply focusing on increasing the vegetable content of your daily diet, you can reduce your total caloric intake without even noticing.

Top 10 ways to eat more vegetables

1 **Order them online** One of the biggest barriers to eating enough fresh produce is having it readily available at home. If you regularly find yourself running out, perhaps it is worth considering a weekly online order from your local veg box scheme or supermarket. Not only is this a cost-effective solution, you are guaranteed seasonal, fresh produce delivered to your door.

2 **Have back ups** Frozen or tinned vegetables are a great back up and can be just as good nutritionally as fresh vegetables if cooked correctly. Steam frozen vegetables lightly and use minimal water, as the vitamins will leach into the water as they are being cooked. Frozen peas, carrots and broccoli can be added to most dishes.

3 **Cut them up immediately** If you cut up vegetables and place them in a bowl in the fridge or middle of the kitchen worktop, you will find the whole family munches on them just because they are there.

4 **Half-the-plate rule** Remember, half your dinner plate should be filled with salad or vegetables – no exceptions.

5 **Add them at lunch** Plain wraps, sandwiches, crackers and sushi are healthy lunch choices but they will not be supplying the amount of bulk from vegetables and salad that you need. Try adding an extra tomato, some cucumber or slices of pepper to your lunch and notice how much more satisfied you feel.

6   **Order extra when eating out** Most restaurants and take-away options including pizza, steak and noodles will not include enough vegetables. Always order extra sides of vegetables to balance your meal nutritionally.

7   **The 5pm munchies** Many of us overindulge in dips, potato crisps and other tasty nibbles at the end of the day, especially as we are preparing dinner. When the late afternoon munchies hit, try snacking on crunchy fresh vegetables with low-fat dip. Not only will you fill yourself up so you don't overeat at dinner, you will have taken care of a couple of portions of vegetables for that day.

8   **Dress them up** Vegetables don't have to be served steamed or soggy with no flavour. There is nothing wrong with baking them in a little olive oil, serving with a light cheese sauce or stir-frying with a small amount of oyster or hoisin sauce for flavour – don't be scared of making them taste good.

9   **Soup or salad?** Studies have shown that starting the meal with a vegetable broth or salad can reduce your calorie intake at the main meal by up to 20 per cent!

10 **Juice it** If all else fails, a vegetable juice made with no fruit is an extremely nutritious addition to the day – so start juicing!

VEGETABLE STACKS

1 butternut squash, peeled and
cut into chunks

2 courgettes

2 tablespoons olive oil

1 large aubergine

1 red pepper

4 large field mushrooms,
stems removed

1 garlic clove, finely chopped

200g asparagus, lightly blanched

100g low-fat feta

Serves 4

1 Preheat the oven to 180°C. Microwave the squash until soft enough to slice, for about 3–5 minutes. Slice the squash and courgettes into thin strips lengthways, brush with some of the oil and place on a baking tray. Bake for 10–20 minutes, or until tender.

2 Cut the aubergine into rounds and pepper into quarters. Brush with the remaining oil and place on a baking tray. Bake for 5–10 minutes, or until tender.

3 Assemble the baked vegetables into 4 stacks on a baking tray. Sit a mushroom on top of each stack. Sprinkle the garlic over the mushroom.

4 Place the stacks back in the oven and bake for about 5–10 minutes, until the mushroom is warmed through.

5 Serve with asparagus spears and crumbled feta.

CHEESY VEGETABLE BAKE

500g cauliflower, cut into small florets

500g broccoli, cut into small florets

1 onion, finely chopped

1 garlic clove, finely chopped

2 slices of low-fat bacon, chopped

1 teaspoon olive oil

¼ cup plain flour

2½ cups (625ml) low-fat milk

¾ cup grated low-fat cheddar cheese

Serves 4–6

1 Preheat the oven to 180°C. Lightly steam the cauliflower and broccoli until just tender. Place in a baking dish.

2 In a saucepan, sauté the onion, garlic and bacon in oil over a medium heat until the onion is soft.

3 Add the flour and cook, stirring, over a low heat for about 1 minute, until smooth. Slowly stir in the milk and bring to the boil, then simmer uncovered for 5–10 minutes, stirring until the sauce is thick. Stir in the cheese.

4 Pour the sauce over the vegetables in the baking dish. Bake for 15–20 minutes or until heated through.

Choose carbs carefully

*'We eat rice, pasta, bread, potatoes and noodles;
too many carbs from too many countries!'*

For many years carbohydrates have been taboo in many weight-loss diets. The theory is that since they are the primary source of fuel for muscle, eliminating them will result in weight loss. However this simplified view of metabolism is not exactly the way things work.

Carbohydrate, one of the four energy-giving nutrients along with protein, fat and alcohol, provides the body with 4 calories of energy per gram. Plant-based foods, including bread, rice, grains, fruit, vegetables and sugars, are all primarily made up of carbohydrates. Once consumed, carbohydrates are broken down into glucose molecules, which are taken to the muscles and brain to be used as fuel. The muscles and liver then store unused glucose in the form of glycogen, which can later be used as energy.

Reducing the intake of carbohydrates will see a short-term reduction in glycogen stores in the muscles. However the body prefers to use glucose as its primary fuel source, so if carbohydrates are being restricted, the body will simply reduce metabolic rate in order to use the available glucose more efficiently. This means the body needs less fuel in order to burn the same amount of calories. Over time, this means you need to eat less food as the muscles need less glucose to do the same amount of work. For example, many individuals who lose large amounts of weight following a low-carb diet put all the weight back on again when they reintroduce carbs. Since most people really do enjoy their carbs, facing a lifetime without them doesn't seem worth it. Instead, being smart about the type of carbs you're eating, how much and at what time is much more achievable.

White bread and rice, processed cakes, biscuits, sweets, fruit juices, soft drinks and potato crisps contain large amounts of processed carbohydrates, which are rapidly digested and offer little nutritionally. These high-GI (glycaemic index) carbs result in a relatively large amount of the hormone insulin being secreted. When the body is exposed to large amounts of insulin over time, weight gain and fat storage results.

Knowing this, the best thing anyone can do to avoid putting their body into this fat-storage mode is to ensure the carbohydrate-rich foods they choose regularly are the best quality, low-GI carbohydrates available. Small slices of dense, wholegrain bread, small portions of wholegrain rice and pasta, grain-based crackers and whole fruit rather than dried or juiced varieties will keep your glucose and insulin working as effectively as possible in your body long-term.

Getting your carb balance right

1   **The more grains the better** The more grains your bread,
    cereal or crackers have, the better they will be for you. Grain-based
    products have some of the lowest GI values, so are digested slowly
    and will leave you feeling full for longer.

2   **Measure your portions** The main issue with rice, pasta, noo-
    dles and breakfast cereal is not the amount of carbohydrate that
    they contain, but how much of them we eat. Aim for just ½–1 cup
    of cooked carbohydrates with your meals.

3   **Go for smaller slices** Have you noticed how much bigger
    slices of bread are getting? Some of the slices are so large they
    don't fit in the toaster. Choose the smallest slices of bread you can
    find and you will be eating up to 20g of carbohydrate less every
    time you eat 2 slices of bread.

4   **Choose your breakfast cereals carefully** Unfortunately
    there are few breakfast cereals on the market that have a low GI.
    Muesli, oats and bran are among the few, which means that the
    popular flakes, rice cereals, honey- and chocolate-flavoured
    varieties need to go.

5   **Always eat carbs and protein together** The GI of
    carbohydrate-containing foods is heavily influenced by what
    foods you eat with them. Aiming for lean protein from meat, fish,
    low-fat dairy or beans with your carbohydrate will naturally lower
    the glycaemic response and help keep you fuller for longer. Good
    examples are wholegrain crackers with low-fat cheese, yoghurt
    with fruit, or rice with tuna.

6   **Be careful with '97% fat free'** In many cases, lowering the fat content means that biscuits, crackers, yoghurts and snack foods have had more sugar added to compensate, which increases their GI value. Such processed foods tend to offer little nutritionally and leave you prone to overeating.

7   **Eat more beans** Legumes including baked beans, chickpeas, kidney beans and lentils have some of the lowest GI ratings. Add to minced meat dishes, salads and stir-fries to bulk up the meal with fibre and protein.

8   **Count the times you eat** The body is designed to eat and then wait at least 2–3 hours before eating again. Constant grazing on milk-based coffees, biscuits and fruit can really disrupt the natural digestive processes and make it difficult to lose weight. Stick to your meals and midmeals and stop snacking in between.

9   **If in doubt, go for brown** If you are unsure of the GI of a food, choosing the brown or wholemeal option is generally better. While not all wholemeal products have a low GI, you will still be getting the benefits of extra protein and fibre.

10 **Be smart with fruit** Of course fruit is a healthy food choice at any time of the day but fruit does have a carbohydrate and calorie load, which means you cannot eat as much as you like. Aim for 2–3 pieces of fruit each day as a snack with yoghurt or nuts, or after meals, and remember the brighter the colour of the fruit, the better it will be for you.

The power of protein

'Protein helps you avoid those sugar highs and lows that leave you prone to overeating.'

Protein, thanks to the numerous Hollywood celebrities who swear by their high-protein regimes, has been the diet buzzword of the decade. Protein is thought to have several benefits for weight control as it is nutrient-rich and keeps you full for longer, and hence more likely to stick to your diet.

Protein contains 4 calories of energy per gram, the same as carbohydrate, and is found in largest amounts in animal products, including meat, chicken, fish and dairy, as well as in soya, nuts and whole grains in smaller amounts. Protein is used for muscle repair, to build skin and hair and to provide essential amino acids that are involved in a number of chemical processes in the body. As proteins are not primarily used as a fuel source, they are also digested after carbohydrates and hence thought to play a powerful role in inducing feelings of satiety or fullness.

POWERFUL PROTEIN CHOICES		
MEAL	**TYPICAL CHOICE**	**HIGHER PROTEIN CHOICE**
Breakfast	Toast with jam	Toast with 1 egg
Midmorning	Fruit	Low-fat cheese and crackers
Lunch	Peanut butter sandwich	50g turkey breast sandwich
Midafternoon	Fruit	Yoghurt and nuts
Dinner	Chicken pad thai	Chicken stir-fry

PROTEIN COUNTER		
PROTEIN SOURCE	**SERVING SIZE**	**PROTEIN PER SERVING (g)**
Beef/pork/lamb	100g	31
Chicken/turkey	100g	28
Seafood	100g	23
Yoghurt	200g	10
Baked beans	1 cup	10
Nuts	50g	10
Milk	250ml	9
Tofu	100g	8
Pasta	1 cup, cooked	8
Egg	1, cooked	7
Rice	1 cup, cooked	7
Cheese	1 slice	5

Meals that contain a significant portion of protein-rich foods in addition to carbohydrates will be digested more slowly than meals or snacks that contain solely carbohydrates. Protein-rich meals and snacks will also tend to offer much more nutritionally, as they are key sources of essential nutrients including iron, zinc, calcium and omega-3 fats.

The common breakfast choices of cereal and toast with jam tend to be low in protein, as do snacks of fruit or snack bars, and lunches of plain sandwiches. Aim to include at least 20g of protein at main meals along with 10–20g of protein at each snack.

Check your good fats

'Every day we need three to four portions of good fats to enhance our cells' ability to burn body fat.'

During the 1980s and 1990s, much time was spent calculating the fat content of everything we ate based on the belief that a low-fat diet would surely result in a low-fat body. The truth is a little more complex than this. Effective fat metabolism (burning) is a complicated process involving a

FAT COUNTER		
FOOD	TOTAL FAT (g)	SATURATED FAT (g)
2 sausages	26	12
1 portion chips	25	12
2 slices cheese	13	8
200g lean mince	14	7
½ avocado	27	6
1 glass full-cream milk	10	6
200g salmon	17	6
10 walnuts	21	1
1 glass low-fat milk	4	1
1 tsp olive oil	5	<1

Remember the average adult needs just 40–60g of (predominantly good) fat per day.

range of different types of fats that come from different foods, in different amounts. As scientists wade through the complex biochemistry, the good news for you is that there are a few key foods that you can include regularly in your diet that will help to achieve an optimal balance of the different types of fat without having to think too much at all.

Fat per gram contains 9 calories of energy. There are two types of fat; saturated and unsaturated. Saturated fat is found predominantly in animal-based and processed foods, is known to increase blood cholesterol and is stored more readily than unsaturated fat. Unsaturated fat, which is found predominantly in plant-based foods, including oils, nuts, seeds and avocados, as well as in oily fish (omega-3), does not increase blood cholesterol and is also more likely to be burnt off than saturated fat.

For a healthy heart and weight control, minimising your intake of saturated fat needs to be the goal for all adults. Dairy food and meat remain the greatest sources of saturated fat in our diet, which is why low-fat milk and lean cuts of meat are recommended by health professionals.

Minimising your saturated fat intake does not mean unsaturated fat can be consumed freely. The average adult needs just 40–60g of fat in total each day. This equates to a portion of oily fish, 10 nuts, a tablespoon of avocado and a teaspoon of olive oil. So if you have been trying to lose weight for some time and are adding a whole avocado to your salad each night, it may simply be a case of too much good fat.

Getting your fat balance right

1. Always choose the leanest meats and low-fat dairy foods.
2. Avoid fatty sausages, salamis and processed meats.
3. Take fish oil capsules.
4. Aim to eat oily fish such as tuna, salmon (see recipe on next page) or sardines three times a week.
5. Eat a handful of nuts each day.
6. Cook with olive or vegetable oil.
7. Choose grain-based bread and crackers.
8. Avoid biscuits, cakes and pastries made using palm oil or hydrogenated vegetable fat.
9. Avoid fast-food outlets that cook with lard or hydrogenated vegetable oils.

SALMON WITH VEGETABLE MASH

Vegetable mash

1 teaspoon olive oil

1 onion, finely sliced

1 small clove garlic, crushed

1 courgette, grated

1 large carrot, grated

½ butternut squash, peeled and diced

2 teaspoons low-fat olive oil spread

4 x 150g salmon fillets, de-boned and skin removed

2 teaspoons wholegrain mustard

¼ cup low-fat sour cream

Serves 4

1 Heat oil in a pan over a medium heat, add onion and garlic. Cook for 2–3 minutes until soft. Stir in grated vegetables and cook for a further 5–8 minutes, or until vegetables are cooked.

2 Place squash in a microwave-safe bowl and add a dash of water. Cover and cook on high for 5 minutes, or until tender.

3 Drain and add cooked squash to vegetable mix and mash until smooth. Stir through olive oil spread and season with salt and pepper to taste. Set aside in a warm place until required.

4 Heat a griddle pan over a medium-high heat. Cook salmon fillets for 3 minutes on one side. Turn over and cook for a further 1–2 minutes for medium rare or until cooked to your liking. Remove and rest for a few minutes.

5 Mix mustard and sour cream together. Top salmon fillets with a dollop of mustard cream. Serve immediately with the mash.

Take your fish oil

'We have not even touched the surface of how important long-chain fats are in our diet.'

Fish oil supplements are capsules made from long-chain fats found in the flesh of deep sea, cold-water fish including tuna, mackerel, salmon and sardines. These fats have a number of health benefits including reducing inflammation, blood pressure and joint pain and swelling.

So what is the benefit for weight loss? Fats get a bad rap for weight loss, but the right balance of fats in our cells helps with metabolism long-term. Saturated fats, found in animal products and processed foods, tend to clog cells up, whereas unsaturated fats make cell walls more fluid, and function more efficiently as a result. We want to keep the intake of saturated fats to a minimum and achieve the right balance of unsaturated fats.

Both poly-unsaturated and mono-unsaturated fats compete to be taken up by our cells. Poly-unsaturated fats, found in salmon, walnuts, soya and linseed, have the most powerful effect on cell walls, so we need to make sure they are not overpowered by the mono-unsaturated fats, which are plentiful in modern diets via almonds, avocado and olive oil. To achieve a good balance of the right fats we need 15–20g of both mono- and poly-unsaturated fats and at least 1g of the long-chain fats found in fish oil. To reach these targets, you need to use olive oil in cooking, eat a handful of walnuts, some oily fish and take 3–6 fish oil capsules a day.

Avoid the diet food

*'I will never be convinced that artificial sweetener
is a better option than sugar.'*

It all sounds so great – diet soft drink, diet yoghurt, diet chocolate, even
diet desserts. Finally we can have all of our favourite foods for fewer
calories and less chance of weight gain. Unfortunately, as is the case with
all things in life, if it seems too good to be true, it usually is.

Diet foods have lower calories than the regular varieties as they have
been sweetened using artificial sweeteners. Artificial sweeteners,
including sucralose, saccharin and aspartame, are synthetically developed
substances that have a similar chemical structure to various sugars but are
up to 500 times sweeter. Such intense sweetness means that only small
amounts of these artificial substances are required to make a food taste
even sweeter than the original food, with fewer calories.

Initially nutritionists reported a number of benefits of consuming less
sugar and calories via artificially sweetened food. But emerging evidence
suggests that consuming large volumes of these foods may actually prime
the brain to crave increasingly sweeter food. It also appears that the brain
may not optimally regulate the calories consumed in products containing
sweeteners, such as diet yoghurt, as they often lack the mouth-feel of
foods with a regular carbohydrate profile. This means we don't feel as
satisfied after eating such products and are likely to eat more.

While swapping to a diet product, especially in the case of soft drink, is a better alternative than choosing the full-sugar version, the truth is that neither product is a healthy component of anyone's diet. While there is nothing wrong with an occasional diet drink, they should not be replacing water as a regular fluid choice.

For those attempting to get back in touch with their body's natural hunger and fullness signals, eliminating the use of sweetener in hot beverages, yoghurts and desserts is a good starting point. Instead of allowing yourself to eat more because it's 'diet', try eating smaller amounts of non-diet foods you enjoy, such as low-fat yoghurt or your favourite dessert. You will find that eating the real thing satisfies you after a smaller amount and you will enjoy it much more. A small amount of sugar that you gradually reduce in your favourite tea or coffee is also a much better option than dosing yourself up on exceptionally sweet drinks all day.

No matter how much we engineer our foods to be lower in calories or richer in flavour, the more natural and clean our food is, the better it will be for us.

Weight-loss superfoods

'Superfoods are only super if we know what the benefits are, how they work and how much of them we should be having.'

'Superfoods' are nutrient-dense foods that also contain powerful antioxidants and promote optimal health long-term. There are a number of key superfoods thought to directly or indirectly support weight loss when used in the right way, at the right time.

CHILLI

The medicinal properties of chilli have been documented for thousands of years. Chilli contains powerful chemicals known as capsaicinoids that increase cell activity and metabolic rate. Adding chilli to your food will give you an extra burn naturally (see recipe on page 49).

GREEN TEA

Green tea is exceptionally high in antioxidants but also thought to slightly increase fat burning. Most recently the polyphenols in green tea have interested neurologists, as they may help to ameliorate neurodegenerative diseases such as dementia. Anecdotal reports suggest that green tea may help to curb sugar cravings that typically follow a meal. Aim for a cup after lunch and dinner, and remember the longer you leave the bag in, the higher the antioxidant content of your cup will be.

SEAWEED

Seaweed is one of the rare foods rich in iodine, which is crucial for optimal thyroid and metabolic functioning. A portion of seaweed 2–3 times each week in sushi or other Asian dishes is a great way to give your body a boost of this important mineral.

SOY AND LINSEED BREAD

Soy and linseed bread is not only low GI, but also a rich source of the long-chain poly-unsaturated fats that most of us need more of. Aim for 2 slices of soy and linseed bread each day.

WALNUTS

Just 10 walnuts provides a massive dose of long-chain poly-unsaturated fats known to optimise the composition of the cell wall, which can allow our fat-burning hormones to work better.

STEAK

Many people eliminate red meat from their diet when they start a weight-loss plan, but lean red meat is among the richest sources of iron, zinc and vitamin B12, which are all crucial for optimal energy production, particularly for active people. Aim for 100g of lean red meat 2–3 times a week as you focus on your weight-loss goals (see recipe on page 49).

CHILLI STEAK

2 x 200g rib-eye steaks

olive oil cooking spray

100g baby spinach leaves

2 medium tomatoes, halved, then sliced

50g low-fat feta, crumbled

15 walnuts

½ red chilli, finely chopped

extra-virgin olive oil to serve

balsamic vinegar to serve

1 Heat a barbecue plate or griddle pan to high. Spray the steaks with cooking spray, then cook for 3–4 minutes on each side for medium, or until done to your liking. Remove from the heat and rest, covered, in a warm place for 5 minutes.

2 In a bowl, gently toss together the spinach, tomatoes, feta, walnuts and chilli. Mix oil and vinegar, then drizzle over steak to serve.

Serves 2

What are you drinking?

'Liquid calories are easily consumed and rarely counted. Water should be the primary fluid of choice for us all.'

The growth of sweetened drinks is a recipe for disaster when it comes to weight control. Liquid calories are easily overconsumed, offer little nutritionally and are hence known as empty calories.

FRUIT JUICE

Freshly squeezed fruit juice seems to epitomise good health. But while fresh fruit is a nutrient-dense snack choice packed with fibre, vitamins and minerals, the concentration of fresh fruit juice means it can be a calorie-dense fluid choice, without the fibre and satiating properties of fresh fruit. Always choose 100 per cent fruit juice, stick to small servings (200ml) and limit your intake to one serving a day to avoid a calorie overload. Better still, try vegetable juices, which contain a third of the calories.

COFFEE

Starting the day with a latte or cappuccino is an indulgence for many people, but large milk-based coffees with added syrup, cream and sugar can contain as much as 500ml of milk, making them more like a meal than a drink. Also slowly sipping sugar and milk-based coffees over many hours is less than ideal metabolically, as it tells the body that you are constantly eating. Aim for no more than 3–4 cups of coffee each day and completely avoid adding sugar or syrups to eliminate as many extra calories as you can.

TEA

Tea is a rich source of antioxidants, and evidence suggests drinking a cup of strong green tea after meals slightly increases metabolic rate. Naturally, all types of tea are best consumed without sugar.

VITAMIN WATER

Vitamin waters have experienced a recent resurgence courtesy of powerful marketing campaigns promising attractive results such as 'vitality' and 'energy'. While these rather expensive waters do contain added vitamins, the reality is that these vitamins are rarely lacking in the average adult's diet and, with up to 6 teaspoons of sugar per bottle, save your money and get your vitamins from fresh fruit and vegetables instead.

SPORTS DRINK

A specially formulated mix of rapidly absorbed carbohydrates and minerals, sports drinks help athletes in their recovery and rehydration after competition. While sports drinks play a role in high-level sport, for those training for less than an hour a day they are generally not necessary.

SOFT DRINK

With up to 9 teaspoons of sugar per 375ml can, in addition to a number of colours and preservatives, soft drink is a calorie-dense, nutrient-poor liquid choice. If you choose to purchase diet varieties, it is useful to be aware that some of the additives used in these drinks have been banned in other countries. (See 'Avoid the diet food' for more information.)

CORDIAL

Cordial, like soft drink, is a nutrient-poor, high-calorie liquid choice and needs to be limited, for both adults and children.

WINE

There is evidence to show that a glass of red wine a night can help to increase the good cholesterol in the bloodstream, but these results are based on drinking just 1 standard-sized glass, not a goblet.

WHAT'S IN YOUR FAVOURITE DRINKS?	
STANDARD SERVING	CALORIES
Regular fruit smoothie (650ml)	360
Grande caramel latte (450ml)	310
Cola drink (600ml)	240
Sports drink (600ml)	185
Large glass of wine (240ml)	170
½ pint standard-strength beer/lager (285ml)	130
Low-fat smoothie (350ml)	120
Vitamin water (500ml)	110
½ pint low-strength beer/lager (285ml)	102
Standard glass of wine (120ml)	85
Small low-fat cappuccino (200ml)	60
Green tea (200ml)	1

BEER

Beer doesn't offer the potential health benefits of spirits and red wine, but you can significantly reduce your caloric intake by choosing low-carb, low-alcohol varieties. Remember it is recommended that women consume no more than 2–3 units of alcohol a day, and men no more than 3–4.

SPIRITS

Spirits, like red wine, contain powerful antioxidants that appear to help increase the levels of good cholesterol in the bloodstream. Spirits do not tend to be overconsumed to the extent that wine and beer are, which can help to control calorie intake. The most important thing in relation to spirits is to watch your mixers – stick to soda water, diet soft drinks or enjoy them on ice to help lower your total caloric intake.

WATER

Water should be the main fluid of choice for all of us and if you are not drinking 1.5–2 litres a day, you are not drinking enough. Not only does keeping hydrated help us (and our skin) to look and feel better, it helps to prevent fatigue, bloating and constipation.

Count the coffees

'If coffee contains milk and sugar, it's a snack.'

We all love our coffee but unless you enjoy it black, it has to be counted as food. If you are enjoying 2–3 coffees with milk and/or sugar before 9am, you have basically been eating for 3 hours and that is why you are not losing weight.

Some people would sacrifice almost anything rather than give up their daily skinny cappuccino. There is nothing wrong with coffee per se; in fact, if consumed in the right amounts, coffee has a number of health benefits, including reduced blood pressure and blood fats, and a reduced risk of developing a number of diseases including some types of cancer. The key thing to know is that the way we drink our coffee and how many times a day we have it is of crucial importance when it comes to weight control.

While a long black contains as few as 2 calories and little to no carbohydrates, a regular skinny latte contains up to 200 calories, with another 15 for every teaspoon of sugar or syrup you add. In fact, if you enjoy two or three of these coffees daily, you are effectively adding an extra 6.5–9lb of body weight over the course of a year.

The best way to enjoy your coffee is with a meal or as a snack – not as an extra. The body needs at least 2–3 hours in between meals without

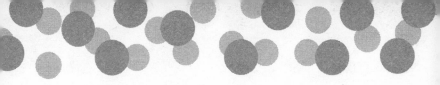

YOUR FAVOURITE BREW	
COFFEE	CALORIES*
Large white	220
Large low-fat latte	130
Small white	120
Small latte	120
Large low-fat cappuccino	100
Small low-fat latte	70
Small low-fat white	70
Small low-fat cappuccino	60

*Remember add an extra 20 calories for every teaspoon of sugar or syrup you add to your favourite brew.

any food stimulus and this includes milk and/or sugar. Black tea or coffee is the best option in between meals. The other important thing to remember with coffee is that no-one needs the large size. A regular size is more than enough, for all of us.

For those who rely on coffee and drink 4 or more cups a day, it may be useful to remember that coffee is a stimulant, increasing central nervous system activity. Relying on such stimulation may mean that there are underlying issues with your diet or lifestyle that need to be addressed. Aim for no more than 3–4 cups of coffee each day and drink more water or herbal tea instead. If you know you need to cut back, it is also important that you wean yourself off gradually so you don't induce the side effects of caffeine withdrawal.

Go 1 month alcohol-free

'An alcohol-free period in the early stages of weight loss is vital.'

Some clients enjoy cheese, others chocolate and others would rather eat bread and water if it meant they could still enjoy a glass of wine at the end of each day.

Alcohol, the fourth energy-containing nutrient after carbohydrate, protein and fat, contains 7 calories of energy per gram, only slightly less than fat, which contains 9 calories per gram. Not only is alcohol relatively high in energy, it is recognised as a toxin by the body and therefore digested before the other three nutrients. This means if you eat when you drink, the body will be so busy burning up the alcohol that it is less likely to get to the food, which is why alcohol and weight gain go hand in hand.

While a small glass of wine contains the same amount of calories as a row of chocolate, the jumbo-sized glasses it is often served in can contain three times this amount. Low-carb and reduced-alcohol varieties are slightly better options, but such a benefit is quickly lost when three or four times the recommended number of drinks is consumed. For most people, one or two standard drinks a night will not cause weight gain per se, the danger comes from the foods we commonly enjoy with them, such as cheese, dips and potato crisps.

In theory, if your caloric intake is below your energy output, even with the inclusion of a glass or two you should still lose weight. Unfortunately in my experience, this is not the case. Perhaps it is because we eat more when we drink, or that we commonly drink at night, or because we have goblet-sized wine glasses. Whatever the reason, if you are serious about weight loss and are a regular drinker, making a decision to go alcohol-free for a month may be the kickstart you need to see a change in the scales, to discover how much you really have been drinking, and to consider if you are really drinking for enjoyment or out of habit.

COMMONLY CONSUMED ALCOHOL	
DRINK	CALORIES
1 pint standard strength beer/lager	260
Large (typical) glass of wine	170
Pre-mixed spirit	165
Bourbon and cola	120
½ pint low-strength beer/lager	102
Small glass of wine	85
Small glass of champagne	85
Glass of low-alcohol wine	75
Bourbon and diet cola	70
Remember we need a total of 1500–2000 calories on average per day.	

To snack or not to snack?

'Being hungry at 3pm is fine, but high-calorie food at this time of day is the worst thing you can do for weight loss.'

Most people have no issue keeping their diet on track during the first half of the day. Breakfast is easy – cereal and fruit, grab yoghurt or coffee midmorning and a healthy salad for lunch. But then the dreaded 3pm munchies hit and you could devour a fridge full of food.

The first step to avoid overeating late in the afternoon is to make sure your lunch contains enough fibre and protein. A light salad or high-GI meal will leave you feeling hungry and unsatisfied a couple of hours after lunch.

THE BEST SNACKS	
SNACK	CALORIES
2 corn thins with 2 tsp peanut butter	190
1 nut-based snack bar	190
4 wholegrain crackers and 2 slices low-fat cheese	165
1 sushi roll	165
10 nuts and 1 piece fruit	140
1 small low-fat latte	140
1 protein shake/bar	140
2 rye crispbreads with cottage cheese and tomato	120
Corn tortilla wrap with ham	120
Natural yoghurt tub with berries	95

The second step is to not let yourself get too hungry, so plan a snack 3 hours after lunch. Eating before you reach absolute starvation will make rational food decisions easier and prevent overeating. Including a snack at this time tends to mean you are less hungry at dinner and only need a small meal. Packaged options like protein- or nut-based bars are easily kept on hand in briefcases or handbags to safely combat the munchies.

The secret to successful snacking is to ensure your choices are portion controlled and take a while to eat. A healthy snack for weight loss needs to keep you full for at least 2 hours and contain a mix of low-GI carbs for energy and protein for fullness. In general they should contain no more than 250 calories, 20–30g of total carbohydrate, 10–20g of protein and <3g of saturated fat per 100g. A trick (that works well for school children too) is to first snack on something that requires a lot of chewing, such as an apple or carrot, followed by one other tasty snack. Then if you're still looking for something else, stick to vegetables, gum or tea.

For mothers, the afternoon is extremely risky when it comes to your food intake. Not only are you likely to be busy ferrying children around, but you are often so busy organising them that you forget that you also need to eat something decent to avoid snacking on rubbish before dinner. Get into a habit of sitting down with the kids for a protein-rich snack at 4pm so you're not ravenous come 5pm.

HEALTHY MUFFINS

½ cup oat bran

1 cup wholemeal flour

1 teaspoon bicarbonate of soda

1½ teaspoons baking powder

½ teaspoon vanilla essence

1 egg

80ml vegetable oil

⅓ cup frozen berries

¼ cup demerara sugar

¼ cup walnuts

Makes 18

1 Preheat the oven to 180ºC. In a large bowl, mix together the oat bran, flour, bicarbonate of soda, baking powder and vanilla.

2 In another bowl, whisk together the egg and oil. Stir in the berries and sugar, then the walnuts. Add to the dry ingredients and mix until just combined.

3 Spoon the batter into greased mini-muffin tins and bake for 20–25 minutes, or until a skewer inserted into a muffin comes out clean.

Nuts once a day

'Remember a portion of nuts is just ten, not half the packet.'

Yes, it is true – nuts are very good for us. In fact, a 30g serving per day is actually linked to weight control long-term. However knowing that nuts are good for us does not mean we can eat them in unlimited volumes. Nuts, like seeds and grains, are relatively high in fat, but the good news is that this fat is predominantly unsaturated, the type of fat that contributes to optimal cell health, helps to regulate a number of hormones and improves good cholesterol levels. Often dieters will keep their total fat intake low and forget the crucial importance of good fats that actually optimise fat metabolism. A portion of 10 nuts each day ensures that we are getting a good dose of poly- and mono-unsaturated fat, protein, fibre and vitamin E.

Aim for a nut-based snack late in the afternoon. Not only will this help to ward off the pre-dinner munchies, but the low-carb content will help to taper your fuel intake towards the second half of the day, which is conducive to weight control.

When it comes to which type, walnuts stand out as the clear winner. Walnuts are known as a 'superfood' as they contain exceptionally high amounts of the long-chain poly-unsaturated fats. For this reason, individuals with high cholesterol can reap many benefits of adding

10 walnuts a day to their diet. The other favourites – peanuts, almonds and cashews – are much higher in mono-unsaturated fats. Their health benefits also tend to be present in a number of commonly eaten foods, including avocado and olive oil.

When purchasing nuts, remember that freshness matters. The fresher the nut, the better its nutrient levels will be. Purchasing your nuts from growers' markets or retailers who have a high turnover will help ensure that you have fresher, better tasting nuts. But remember portion control is key. If you buy your nuts in large bags, repackage them immediately into portion-controlled servings.

HOW MUCH FAT IS IN NUTS?				
SERVING OF 10	TOTAL FAT (g)	POLY FAT (g)	MONO FAT (g)	SAT FAT (g)
Walnuts	21	15	4	1
Macadamias	15	<1	12	2
Almonds	7	2	4	<1
Cashews	7	1	5	1
Peanuts	4	1	2	1

CHICKEN AND WALNUT SALAD

1 cup shredded cooked chicken

1 large celery stick, diced

1 small carrot, grated

1 green apple, diced

⅓ cup toasted walnuts, roughly chopped

Dressing

1 tablespoon mayonnaise

2 teaspoons fresh lime juice

1 In a bowl, gently toss chicken, vegetables, apple and nuts together.

2 To make the dressing, mix mayonnaise and lime juice, pour over salad and mix through.

Serves 1

Never leave the house without two vegetables

'Remember if it's in front of you, you will eat it.'

It may seem like a strange suggestion but always having a vegetable-based snack with you – whether it be a carrot, some celery sticks or baby tomatoes – means you are more likely to get the number of vegetable portions that you need each day and also always have a filling snack on hand.

Many of us eat too many calories simply because we do not eat enough of the low-calorie foods to bulk up our diet and keep us full. Meals and snacks we choose on the run often contain a small volume of vegetable bulk, but it is exceptionally easy to add. Munching on a carrot or celery, or adding tomatoes or rocket to crackers will bulk up your diet and leave you craving fewer snacks.

The 'two vegetables' rule will become as easy as remembering to grab your keys as you leave the house. You will need to purchase larger volumes of vegetables and salad each week so you always have supplies on hand. Remember, if it's in front of you, you will eat it.

Know the best treats

'There is nothing wrong with eating some chocolate –
it's eating the whole block that brings things undone.'

Crisps, chocolate, cheese and cakes – imagine how easy it would be to manage your weight without the 4 Cs? The danger with these tasty treats is that they are not only very high in fat, but they are also very easy to overeat. A block of chocolate while watching TV, a 200g packet of crisps at a barbecue, a round of brie with a glass of wine and you have consumed a massive amount of both fat and calories.

There is growing evidence that the complex mix of sugar and fat found in chocolate, ice-cream, cakes and pastries may actually prime the brain to seek more and more of this type of food. Such intense flavours light up reward centres in the brain, which over time encourages the brain to look for such stimulation again. Eating these foods reinforces the brain's cravings rather than satisfying them.

We have often been programmed from an early age to strongly desire the 4 Cs. Many of us will have powerful memories of parents hiding treat foods, rewarding good behaviour with chocolate and only having crisps and cake on special occasions. These restrictions programme our brain to seek reward from these foods and strongly desire what we have not been freely allowed. This reaction tends to be worse the more restricted the food has been. This is why some children will overeat at birthday parties – they have been constantly deprived of certain foods so have not learnt how to regulate their intake when they are readily available.

Ideally by the time we reach adulthood, we will have learnt to manage ourselves around these types of food. We would be able to keep a block of chocolate in the fridge and enjoy a row at a time, or not eat the whole packet of biscuits simply because they are there. For many of us, this early programming is too strong, and limiting our exposure to these tempting treats is the best way to control ourselves until we break the habit.

If you struggle with portions, buying blocks of chocolate or large tubs of ice-cream is a recipe for disaster. Buy portion-controlled options only, or buy them only as you need them if you really struggle. Incorporating your favourite foods into your daily diet is the best way to develop a sustainable model of eating without negative effects on weight control.

KNOWING THE 4 Cs		
TREATS	CALORIES	FAT (g)
250g block of chocolate	1300	68
1 slice of chocolate cake	310	17
1 slice of banana bread	300	20
50g packet of potato crisps	260	17
1 row of chocolate	150	8
¼ round of brie	100	9
30g feta cheese	80	7

Low-calorie treats

2 squares of dark chocolate
1 individually wrapped chocolate
1 chocolate biscuit
1 low-fat hot chocolate
1 low-fat ice-cream on a stick
1 mango ice-cream bar
1 muesli cookie
2 rye crispbreads and 1 slice of low-fat cheese
2 corn thins with low-fat cream cheese
2 tablespoons of thick yoghurt with berries

Breakfast success

'There is no point even trying to lose weight unless you are eating a protein-rich breakfast before 8am.'

Despite strong evidence that breakfast helps boost metabolic rate and fat loss, there are still many of us who do not get our first meal of the day right. Choosing high-GI breakfast options such as sugary cereals, raisin toast or bagels, or skipping breakfast altogether can leave you more likely to overeat during the rest of the day and ultimately lead to long-term weight gain. Breakfast skippers often claim they feel ill if they eat early. This is merely a result of programming the body not to look for food until much later in the day and will subside once you start slowly reintroducing small breakfasts. The good news is that for even those completely turned off by the thought of cereal and milk, a healthy breakfast can be simple once you know a few tricks of food digestion and metabolism.

The first thing to keep in mind is that the body's digestive hormones are programmed according to a 24-hour circadian rhythm. This means that after an overnight fast of 8–12 hours without food, the body is ready to refuel with energy from carbohydrates. Failing to refuel for an extra 3–4 hours by putting off breakfast until 10 or 11am slows the metabolic rate as the body senses starvation and acts to conserve energy. It even seems the bigger the better when it comes to our breakfast choices. A recent paper published in the *International Journal of Obesity* found that individuals on a weight-loss diet lost twice as much body fat when they consumed half of their daily calories at breakfast.

It's crucial for weight loss to get the right balance of key nutrients at breakfast that will satisfy you for 2–3 hours and promote fat burning rather than fat storage. Choices that have a high carbohydrate load relative to protein such as toast with a spread, large helpings of cereal, raisin toast, muffins and white breads leave you vulnerable to high insulin levels and hunger throughout the morning. Better choices include wholegrain toast with eggs (see recipe on page 71), low-fat cheese, baked beans or protein-based drinks. Such options will help you regulate your appetite, maintain optimal energy and support your weight control long-term.

Top 10 breakfast options

1 1–2 poached eggs on 1–2 slices of wholegrain toast

2 130g tin of baked beans on 1 slice of wholegrain toast

3 ⅓ cup oats + 1 cup low-fat milk

4 Protein shake or liquid-meal drink

5 Egg breakfast wrap

6 ⅓ cup muesli + thick yoghurt + fruit

7 ¾ cup wholegrain breakfast cereal + low-fat milk

8 Protein bar or breakfast bar

9 Low-fat latte + 1 piece of fruit

10 Smoked salmon on 1–2 slices of wholegrain toast

QUICK BEANS
AND SCRAMBLED EGGS

Beans

1 tablespoon light olive oil

1 onion, finely sliced

2 garlic cloves, crushed

4 vine-ripened
tomatoes, finely diced

1 cup cooked cannellini beans
or other white beans

Scrambled eggs

2 eggs

2 egg whites

2 tablespoons low-fat milk

olive oil cooking spray

2 tablespoons chopped
flat-leaf parsley

2 slices of wholegrain toast

1 To make the beans, heat the oil in a saucepan. Add the onion and garlic and sauté over a medium heat for 2 minutes, or until golden. Stir in the tomatoes and beans and cook for 7 minutes, or until the tomato has reduced and thickened. Keep warm.

2 To make the scrambled eggs, whisk together the eggs, egg whites and milk in a small bowl. Spray a non-stick frying pan with cooking spray, heat gently over a low heat and pour the egg mix into the pan. Stir with a wooden spoon until the egg is just set. Sprinkle with parsley.

3 Serve the scrambled eggs with the beans and wholegrain toast.

Serves 2

your lunch balance right

'If you are craving sugar at 4pm, you haven't eaten properly at lunchtime.'

After years of reading nutrition information you know that breakfast is important, and that you need to eat more vegetables. You also know that a tuna salad is a good choice for lunch – or is it? What we choose for lunch as well as the time we eat it can have a big impact on the way we eat and feel for the remainder of the day. This is a nutrition area surprisingly overlooked, particularly by busy people. Getting the balance right is very easy, as is preparing a tasty yet nutritious lunch which may be slightly more appealing than your usual but rather dull tuna and salad.

SOME GOOD-QUALITY CARBS

The first component of a nutritionally balanced lunch is a portion of low-GI carbs. For all the carb-phobics out there who try and keep their intake as low as possible, remember that carbs are the main fuel for the muscle. Choosing to starve your muscles of carbs throughout the day is more likely to leave you craving them later in the afternoon. A much better approach is to include a portion of low-GI carbs at lunch and then keep your intake of energy-dense carbs such as biscuits, cakes and bread lighter during the second half of the day.

Tinned beans or sweetcorn, wholemeal pasta or brown rice (see salad recipe on page 75), wholegrain crackers or 1–2 slices of dense grain, flat or sourdough bread are all good lunch choices. Naturally more active people require more carbs throughout the day than those less active. As a rough guide, a female who exercises for an hour each day will need roughly 1 cup of rice or pasta or 2 slices of bread. A more active, large male will require more; a more sedentary person less.

A SERVING OF NUTRIENT-RICH PROTEIN

A couple of slices of ham is not enough. We need a good-sized helping of lean protein included in our lunch choice to help avoid the 3–4pm munchies. Tins of tuna or salmon, a palm-sized piece of chicken breast or lean red meat, an egg or tofu are nutrient-rich options that will ensure your salad, sandwich or sushi will keep you full throughout the afternoon. Always keep a couple of tins of tuna handy in your desk drawer to add to salads or vegetables, or plan ahead and make enough dinner to give you tasty leftovers if you struggle with eating protein in your lunch.

MORE VEGETABLES OR SALAD THAN YOU THINK!

The most common mistake healthy eaters make is forgetting how much salad and vegetable bulk they need in their lunch. A few lettuce leaves or tomato slices is not enough – ideally you need at least 3–4 different vegetables with your lunch to give you the fibre, vitamins, minerals and bulk that will keep you full throughout the afternoon. Carry hard vegetables such as carrots and celery with you to munch on, or prepare an extra green salad the night before to enjoy with your regular sandwich, soup or sushi.

WORST LUNCH CHOICES		
FOOD CHOICE	**CALORIES**	**FAT (g)**
Burger and fries	880	40
Pad thai	810	46
Chicken and avocado on ciabatta	760	54
Quiche	475	30
Stir-fried chicken and rice	475	30
Pesto chicken salad	475	35

TOP LUNCH CHOICES		
FOOD CHOICE	**CALORIES**	**FAT (g)**
Leftover pasta with meat and vegetable sauce	330	7
2 tuna sushi rolls	330	6
Wholegrain crackers with salmon and rocket	285	6
Chicken and salad wrap	285	6
Frittata and salad	285	7
Tuna, beans and salad	240	7

BROWN RICE SALAD

Rice salad

½–¾ cup cooked brown rice

1 cup roasted diced pumpkin

1 small red pepper, finely chopped

2 handfuls baby spinach leaves

½ cup walnuts

50g low-fat feta, crumbled

Garlic-lemon dressing

1 tablespoon extra-virgin olive oil

1 garlic clove

2 teaspoons lemon juice

1 In a bowl, mix together the rice, vegetables, walnuts and feta.

2 In a separate bowl, whisk together the dressing ingredients.

3 Drizzle the dressing over the salad and serve.

Serves 1

Halve your dinner

'Most of us eat so much during the day that we don't really need dinner.'

Halving the size of your dinner is a powerful weight-loss tool, but it doesn't have to be as dramatic as it seems. Simply reducing the size of your protein portion and aiming for a much larger portion of vegetables or salad is all you need to do, especially if you regularly find yourself eating late. Alternatively swap your dinner for soup a few nights a week to reduce your caloric intake while still enjoying a hearty meal.

Up to 30 per cent of lunch and dinner meals are eaten away from the home and restaurant meals have significantly more calories and fat than home-prepared options. To help counter this, aiming for a very light dinner the rest of the week is an easy way to strike a balance.

MAKING GOOD DINNER CHOICES			
REGULAR MEAL	CALORIES	SMART SWAP	CALORIES
Spaghetti bolognaise	400	3 meatballs and salad	200
Chicken schnitzel	420	100g grilled chicken breast	190
Roast dinner	610	100g grilled steak and salad	200
Pad thai	420	Thai beef salad	260

Cut your carbs at night

'Does cutting out the heavy carbs at night help with weight loss? Yes.'

No studies have clearly shown that eliminating carbohydrate-rich foods including bread, rice, pasta and potato at the evening meal is specifically effective in supporting weight loss. However in my clinical experience, in which I have seen hundreds of clients of all ages, backgrounds and fitness levels, cutting back on carbs at night does help weight loss, at least initially. But such a weight-loss technique cannot be used long-term.

While cutting back on carbs is a good theory, in practice such a technique is often rendered useless as carbs are replaced by other high-calorie, high-fat foods, such as larger servings of meat or dessert after the meal. The ultimate goal of weight loss is to get your body to burn its fuel more efficiently, so ideally we want to use our muscles more to burn more fuel. Using our muscles more means we need more carbs to allow them to function at their best and burn fat effectively, so the trick here is to be mindful of portions sizes and the type of carbohydrates you reintroduce into your diet.

Generally speaking, energy-dense carbs can be eliminated from the evening meal for 2–4 weeks or until a bit of weight is lost. Once this has occurred, try reintroducing half a cup of cooked carbs to your evening meal and steadily increase to a healthy amount that keeps you energised for training. A woman who trains an hour each day will require roughly ½–1 cup of cooked carbohydrate at night to keep weight stable. A lean male who trains for an hour a day will generally need between 1–2 cups of cooked carbohydrate with his evening meal.

WARM LAMB SALAD

150g packet or 3 cups of assorted lettuce leaves

1 cucumber, chopped

1 red pepper, chopped

4 plum tomatoes, chopped

200g pumpkin, roasted and diced

100g low-fat feta, chopped

400g lean lamb fillets

1 tablespoon olive oil

tzatziki yoghurt dip to serve

1 In a bowl, gently toss together vegetables and feta.

2 Finely slice the lamb fillets and brush all over with the oil. Sear lightly in a very hot wok or frying pan until medium–rare.

3 Arrange the lamb over the vegetables, drizzle with tzatziki and serve.

Serves 4

Know your quick and easy meals

'When you come home tired, you can order Thai, or throw a quick, nutritious meal together without excess calories.'

Life is busy and it's only likely to become more so. Less perceived time for food preparation tends to mean more takeaways, and more calories as a result. For this reason, knowing some quick and easy meals you can throw together in a few minutes is a crucial part of eating well for the larger part of the week (see recipes on pages 82–4).

When meals are prepared in a hurry, high-carb, low-vegetable options tend to fill our plates. Noodles, pasta or toast are common favourites, but we need both a vegetable and lean protein component if we are to keep the nutrition up and the calories down. Here are the best supermarket foods you can have at home for quick meals on the run.

FROZEN FISH

The health benefits of eating fish regularly are well publicised, but it can be challenging to have fresh fish available, or to get the kids to eat it! The good news is there is an increasing number of frozen fish varieties that are both nutritious and taste good. Check nutrition labels and choose varieties that contain less than 10g of total fat per 100g.

FROZEN VEGETABLES

Yes, frozen vegetables are still good choices nutritionally, if you don't overcook them. Another benefit is that unlike tinned varieties, frozen vegetables do not contain added salt. Remember, the more colourful the vegetables, the better they will be for you. Try steaming or stir-frying them to retain as much nutritional value as possible.

TOMATO PASTA SAUCE

Whether you add it to pasta or cook your meat or seafood in it, tomato pasta sauce is lycopene-rich and can be added to many meals. Salt-reduced options are the best.

TINNED TUNA

Another pantry staple, tinned tuna can also be added to pasta, a jacket potato, bread or crackers for a tasty, protein-rich, nutritious meal option. While low-fat varieties of tuna may appear to be better nutritionally, remember you get a significant amount of omega-3 fat from fish, so low-fat options may not be the best choice.

LOW-FAT MOZZARELLA

A sprinkle of cheese on top of the right mix of foods can make a meal – and mozzarella has significantly less fat than parmesan and cheddar cheeses. Add to jacket potatoes, grilled chicken or veal, or homemade pizza for a calcium hit minus the fat.

TASTY MINCE

2 teaspoons olive oil

1 onion, chopped

1 garlic clove, diced

500g extra-lean mince

100g salt-reduced
tomato paste

200g tin of diced tomatoes

2–3 cups mixed
frozen vegetables

sprinkle of mozzarella and
green salad to serve

1 Warm the oil in a frying pan.
Add the onion and garlic and
cook for 2 minutes. Add the
mince and cook until browned.

2 Add the tomato paste, tomatoes
and vegetables and simmer
over a medium heat for 15–20
minutes, until cooked through.

3 Serve with a sprinkle of
mozzarella and a large green
salad.

Serves 4

SALMON PASTA

2 cups wholemeal pasta

180g tin red salmon

100g natural yoghurt

2 tomatoes, chopped

green salad to serve

Serves 4

1 Cook the pasta in a saucepan
of boiling salted water until
just tender. Drain and return
to the pan.

2 Add the salmon, yoghurt and
tomato and gently mix. Gently
reheat until warmed through,
about 3–5 minutes. Serve with a
salad.

COURGETTE OMELETTE

olive oil cooking spray

2 eggs, lightly beaten

½ small courgette, finely grated

4 mushrooms, chopped

1 tomato, diced

1 red pepper, diced

50g low-fat ham, sliced

¼ cup low-fat grated cheese

Serves 1

1 Place a non-stick frying pan over a medium heat. Spray with cooking spray, then add the egg and swirl to coat the base of the pan.

2 Sprinkle the egg with the remaining ingredients. Cook for 2 minutes, or until the egg has set, then turn the omelette over and cook the other side.

3 Remove from the pan and set aside to cool slightly. Roll the omelette up, cut into slices and serve.

PRAWNS AND COURGETTE

1 small courgette, sliced

10 raw prawns, shelled and deveined

4–5 mushrooms, sliced

½ cup tomato pasta sauce

50g low-fat feta

Serves 1

1 Place a non-stick frying pan over a medium heat. Add the courgette and sauté until just cooked through.

2 Add the prawns and cook, stirring, until they are translucent, for about 2–3 minutes.

3 Stir in the mushroom and pasta sauce and simmer until heated through, for about 3–5 minutes. Crumble the feta over and serve.

STUFFED POTATO

1 potato, with skin on, scrubbed well

100g tin of tuna in oil, drained

1 small tomato, chopped

½ pepper, chopped

¼ cup grated low-fat cheddar cheese

Serves 1

1 Preheat the oven to 180ºC. Microwave the potato in its skin until tender, for about 5 minutes on medium.

2 Slice the potato open and fill with the tuna, tomato and pepper. Sprinkle with the cheese.

3 Bake for 5–10 minutes, or until the cheese has melted.

Soup it up

'Who would have thought that a humble bowl of soup could offer so many weight-loss benefits?'

A dietitian always has tricks in her or his toolbox. My favourite is a recipe that can relatively quickly shift fluid, leaving you feeling lighter and in a good place psychologically to continue with your weight-loss regime.

Vegetable-based soups have an extremely high nutrient content, are very low in calories and provide bulk to prevent you feeling hungry and deprived as you would using meal-replacement shakes. Studies show that enjoying a broth-based soup before a meal can reduce caloric intake for the remainder of the meal by 20 per cent. As favoured by the skinny French, soups that have a base of leeks, onions and/or celery (see recipe on page 86) are particularly high in the mineral potassium. Potassium helps rid the body of the excess fluid many of us carry thanks to a high-salt diet and lack of activity, but dropping as little as 500g, even if it is just fluid, can make us feel lighter and leaner instantly.

For those wanting a more intense regime or short-term results, vegetable soup can replace two meals a day for 5–7 days without negative side effects.

CHICKEN AND VEGETABLE SOUP

2 skinless chicken breast fillets, diced

4 cups (1 litre) reduced-salt chicken stock

1 tablespoon vegetable oil

2 leeks, white part only, finely sliced

2 carrots, diced

2 celery sticks, diced

3 garlic cloves, crushed

6 cups or 200g young green salad leaves, such as watercress, rocket, sorrel and baby spinach, finely chopped

3 tablespoons fresh pesto

Serves 6

1 Place the chicken in a saucepan and pour in just enough stock to cover. Poach gently for 10 minutes, or until the chicken is just cooked. Set aside to cool.

2 Heat the oil in a large saucepan. Add the leek and gently sauté until soft, for about 2 minutes. Stir in the carrot, celery and garlic.

3 Strain the chicken-poaching stock through a fine sieve, then add to the vegetables with the remaining stock. Simmer for 10 minutes. Stir in the greens and simmer for a further 10 minutes.

4 Shred the chicken and add it to the soup. Stir in the pesto and season to taste with plenty of freshly ground black pepper.

Learn to love salads

'Want to slash your calories at dinner?
Just add a salad – it's that simple.'

If you consider that simply eating a large green salad before you tuck into your dinner can reduce your total energy intake by as much as 120 calories, it may be worth chopping up a few extra greens each week. The humble lettuce not only adds bulk to your diet and helps you to eat less, but it is extremely low in calories. Adding extra salad to both your lunch and evening meal will improve the nutritional profile of your diet in general.

Salads can be great lunch choices but it's useful to know that they can also be packed with a lot of fat, particularly if you add nuts, cheese, dressing

POPULAR SALAD CHOICES		
SALAD	CALORIES	FAT (g)
Chicken caesar salad	520	30
Chicken pesto salad	475	36
Greek salad	285	26
Vietnamese chicken salad	285	10
Thai beef salad	260	9
Pumpkin and pine nut salad	240	20
Green salad with dressing	120	10

and avocado. For this reason, including no more than one high-fat salad ingredient is crucial if you want to reap the benefits.

MAKING THE PERFECT SALAD MEAL

Step 1 – Salad greens Whether you choose cos lettuce, rocket or baby spinach, follow this mantra: the darker the leaves, the better they are for you. Salad leaves are rich sources of fibre, vitamins C and K and generally form the base of a salad that will help to keep you full for a number of hours after eating it.

Step 2 – Plenty of brightly coloured vegetables The more you include, the better the salad will be for you – carrots, cucumber, celery, tomatoes, beetroot, pumpkin and peppers. If you find yourself throwing out too much fresh produce, try making one large salad base each week and adding the wetter items, such as tomatoes, later. This way you always have some salad ready to go and can even add it to sandwiches, wraps and crackers as extra fillers throughout the day.

Step 3 – Carbs for energy A plain salad enjoyed at lunch without any bread, crackers or other forms of carbohydrate may appear to be the most healthy, calorie-controlled option but remember that not eating adequate carbs throughout the day can leave you feeling unsatisfied and more likely to binge later in the afternoon. Adding a small amount of low-GI carbohydrate to your salad in the form of sweet potato, sweetcorn or beans, or enjoying the salad with a slice of wholegrain bread or crackers will perfectly complement your lunchtime salad.

Step 4 – Lean protein for nutrition A small tin of tuna or salmon, 1–2 eggs or a palm-sized portion of lean meat or chicken are not only a filling component of your salad but also have much to offer nutritionally. Protein foods are rich sources of iron, zinc, vitamin B12 and omega-3 fats. Remember, the less processed the better, and if you choose tuna in olive oil, make sure that you drain off the extra oil to avoid a fat overload.

Step 5 – Added fats Salad dressings, nuts and cheese may all be tasty additions to your salad but they are high-fat choices and can quickly turn your healthy salad into a calorie overload if you're not careful. Aim for just one of these additions to your salad and remember that olive oil and walnuts are the two best high-fat additions due to their optimal fat profile.

HALOUMI SALAD

500g butternut squash, peeled and chopped

250g punnet of cherry tomatoes

olive oil cooking spray

100g low-fat haloumi cheese, sliced

150g baby spinach

Honey-mustard dressing

1 tablespoon wholegrain mustard

1 tablespoon honey

a dash of balsamic vinegar

2 tablespoons extra-virgin olive oil

Serves 4

1 Preheat the oven to 180ºC. Spread the squash in a baking tin and roast for 15–20 minutes, or until tender. Add the tomatoes and roast for a further 5 minutes, or until the tomatoes start to collapse. Place in a bowl.

2 Warm a non-stick frying pan over medium heat. Coat pan with cooking spray, then add the haloumi and fry briefly on both sides until lightly golden. Add to the roasted vegetables with the spinach and gently toss.

3 In a small bowl, whisk together the dressing ingredients and drizzle over the salad. Serve with grilled lamb or chicken, or as a meal with chickpeas.

TIP Always look for low-fat haloumi, as the full-fat option can contain 20+ grams of fat per serving.

Embrace a sugar detox

*'If you constantly crave sweet foods,
it may be time to do a sugar detox.'*

You know the drill: you start the day with a caramel latte, are hanging out for some banana bread at morning tea and feel like you are going to die at 3 or 4pm if you don't get your hands on some diet soft drink and a chocolate bar. If this sounds even remotely familiar, you may need a sugar detox to take control of your tastebuds and eating habits.

From the time we are given our first taste of mashed banana or custard as babies we are embracing a reward system that programmes us to seek pleasure from sweet foods. It doesn't matter if you get your sweet fix from diet yoghurt, fruit, low-fat banana bread, low-calorie biscuits or low-fat dessert, the fact that you are constantly searching for sweet taste sensations is the real issue. Until you alter this drive, you are going to be constantly craving and seeking out more and more sweet foods to satisfy the desire.

Generally it will take at least 2–3 days without any sweet food for you to no longer be searching for it. This means you're going to have to work through a mini-detox and possibly some withdrawal symptoms, including headaches, cravings, irritability and fluctuating blood sugar levels. As you submit to this process, keep in mind that the need for sweet foods can be shifted by tasting savoury and salty foods, anything that shifts the palate.

SUGARS IN FOOD		
FOOD	CALORIES	TEASPOONS OF SUGAR
200ml low-fat fruit yoghurt	170	5
1 cup Cheerios	110	2
Glass of cordial	100	5
2 plain biscuits	80	3
2 Weight Watchers biscuits	36	2
2 jelly snakes	40	2
1 tbsp tomato sauce	20	1

Useful foods at this time include those with strong mint flavours, green tea or savoury proteins.

The good news is that once you've detoxed from sweet foods, over time you'll notice that you get the same amount of pleasure from naturally sweet foods like yoghurt and fruit as you once did from cakes and biscuits. You will also need far less of the very sweet foods to get the same hit you once needed. Ultimately this means less high-calorie sweet food will be entering your mouth, which ultimately means less weight long-term and a new you who is no longer controlled by your sugar cravings.

Are you having any extras?

'All the hidden extras really do add up.'

A spread of margarine here, a dollop of sauce there and before you know it you have an extra 200 calories a day, which is the difference between weight loss and not. There is no denying that these little extras make our food taste better, but as these small additions gradually become larger, they really add up.

Let's start with spreads. Butter or margarine contains at least 30 calories per teaspoon. Unless you are being mindful you are likely to be using far more than you think and in many cases just adding calories rather than flavour. High-calorie spreads including nut pastes, jam, honey and chocolate spreads are all recipes for disaster when it comes to extra calories. Such options offer little nutritionally, and they are extras we can easily do without once we are basing our food choices around a good carb and protein balance.

Sugar in tea and coffee is another trap to avoid. What should be a level 5g teaspoon is more likely to be heaped and the more you have, the more you want. Swap to sugar cubes or wean off altogether.

Avocado is another addition we take for granted. The ideal 20g portion is more likely to become half the fruit added to salads and sandwiches rather than the thin spread or light scattering it should be.

Sauces are the next issue. Soy, oyster, tomato, barbecue – you are adding about 10–20 calories per teaspoon. Start to measure your portions so you know how much you are really using.

Olive oil can quickly add up too. While celebrity chefs heartily pour litres of the stuff into their cooking, if you consider that just 1 teaspoon of oil contains more than 40 calories, you can see how easy it is to go overboard. Use spray oils where possible and measure your quantities when adding oil to pastas or salad.

EXTRAS CALORIE COUNTER		
EXTRA	CALORIES	FAT (g)
1 tbsp peanut butter	155	13
¼ avocado	130	14
1 tbsp jam	70	0
1 syrup shot in coffee	65	0
1 tsp olive oil	40	4
1 tsp margarine	35	4
1 tbsp sweet chilli sauce	25	<1
1 tbsp tomato sauce	20	0
1 tsp sugar	17	0

Go smaller

'We eat far more than we think we do.'

Serving sizes have become a whole lot bigger. Soft drinks now come in 600ml bottles as the norm, potato crisps in 100g packets and even the average slice of bread won't fit in a regular toaster. Yet while servings are increasing, we are moving less so actually need fewer calories to fuel our muscles. It's not difficult to see how weight gain is almost inevitable.

Behavioural research has repeatedly shown that people will eat what is in front of them. For example, if you have chocolates on your desk in a glass container instead of a ceramic container, you will eat double the number simply because you can see them. You are not weak, you are just human.

A realistic weight-loss trick that allows you to enjoy your favourite foods while controlling your weight is to simply monitor your portion sizes, at every meal, every day. Reducing caloric intake gradually over time and maintaining the reduction is ultimately the trick to long-term weight control.

So how can you get a firm grasp of your own portion distortion? Let's start with breakfast. Measure just ¾ cup of breakfast cereal and serve it in a small shallow bowl, rather than a soup-style bowl. Choosing smaller slices of bread and smearing no more than a teaspoon of butter on your toast means you will have saved yourself more than 50 calories. That may not seem like much but if you save this amount of energy every day, that is more than 250 calories per week, or almost 4.5lb of body weight over the course of a year.

Next is your choice of coffee cup size. Large coffees contain as many calories as a meal, yet few of us count them as such. Generally coffee shops will offer regular-sized cups that contain at least 250 calories more than small cups. Always ask for small coffees.

Then onto morning tea. Large packets of potato crisps, biscuits, cheese, nuts and sweets are setting you up to fail. Individual-sized portions of yoghurt, cheese and crackers are convenient ways to make sure you do not over serve yourself. If you are craving something sweet, remember that the most pleasure is derived from your first few mouthfuls of food so just a third or half a slice of cake should be more than enough to satisfy any cravings.

At lunchtime remember that sandwiches purchased from sandwich bars provide double the amount of calories you really need from your lunch, so you may only need to eat half a large sandwich with a piece of fruit to satisfy you. If you are making your lunch, a few crackers or a slice of flat bread is often all you need to keep you full for another 2–3 hours. Other high-risk foods that tend to be overeaten during the day include nuts (10 is a serving), avocado (¼ is a serving) and salad dressings (you only need a teaspoon).

For your evening meal, try weighing your portions of meat to grasp how much you are actually having. Women will need just 100–150g and men 150–200g of lean meat, chicken or fish. Helpings of salmon and steak can often be double this size.

Finally your treats at night – tubs of ice-cream and blocks of chocolate are asking for trouble. If you do enjoy a sweet treat at night, always look for portion-controlled servings and stick to less than 100 calories.

SIMPLE CHANGES, HUGE CALORIE REDUCTION

The table below is a reminder of how some simple changes can have a massive impact on calorie intake over the course of a year. These figures are based on estimates of consumption frequency over a week.

CALORIE SAVING SWAPS			
SWAP	FOR	CALORIES SAVED	BODY FAT EQUIV. /YEAR
1 tbsp oil	1 tsp oil	125	4.5lb
200g meat	150g meat	75	4lb
1 large slice bread	1 small slice bread	40	2.5lb
Margarine on toast	Olive oil spread on toast	35	4.5lb
1 cup cereal	¾ cup cereal	25	0.5lb
Tea with milk	Herbal tea	10	1.5lb
1 heaped tsp sugar	1 cube sugar	5	3.5lb

Choose hard foods

'The more chewing you have to do,
the better the food is likely to be for you.'

If you had been around hundreds of thousands of years ago you would have had to chase your own dinner, scrounge for edible plants and chew through tough meat to survive. Fast-forward to the present day and many foods barely need chewing at all. Bread is fluffy, meat is minced, grains are ground right down – food on the whole is soft and mushy.

The body burns significantly more calories digesting hard, unprocessed food than softer processed foods. You will expend more energy digesting a steak than you will the same type and amount of minced meat. Fillets of meat, dense grain bread, oats or muesli, raw vegetables, nuts – these are all foods the body has to work hard to break down. White bread, minced meat, peanut butter and refined cereals have more calories, are eaten (and overeaten) more easily and don't keep us full.

Chewing is a good guide. Ideally we need to chew each mouthful many times in order to slow the digestive process and allow the body to register that it's full. In fact, the simple act of slowing down the eating process has been shown to reduce the caloric intake at a meal by as many as 100 calories. So if in doubt, when choosing foods, the harder the better.

BEEF AND MANGETOUT STIR-FRY

500g lean rump steak

1 tablespoon brown sugar

2 tablespoons sunflower oil

250g mangetouts

2 large carrots, thinly sliced on the diagonal

2 red peppers, cut into chunks

⅓ cup (80ml) oyster sauce

2 tablespoons soy sauce

2 cups steamed brown rice to serve

1 Rub the beef all over with the sugar and half the oil and cut into thin strips.

2 Heat a wok and lightly stir-fry the beef and transfer to a plate.

3 Heat the remaining oil in the wok. Quickly stir-fry the vegetables in the oyster sauce and soy sauce until just tender.

4 Return the beef to the wok. Toss until well combined and heated through. Serve immediately, with steamed brown rice.

Serves 4

Quality over quantity

'Think quality over quantity when it comes to food and you'll never go wrong.'

Enjoying good food is an important pleasure in life – the first bite of a scrumptious dessert, fresh mango juice running down your chin, the first sip of a great pinot. But how many times throughout the day do you eat for no such enjoyment? The cheap, dry birthday cake at work, half a piece of cold toast from the kids' breakfast? All less-than-perfect food experiences that are better skipped both from a taste and calorie perspective.

There is absolutely nothing wrong with enjoying good-quality food, including chocolates, desserts and restaurant meals, in the right amounts if you really feel like them, but spending your calories on poor-quality, high-calorie foods simply because they're there is just a waste of calories. Remember the most pleasure is gained from the first couple of mouthfuls. This means that generally just a spoon or so of that chocolate soufflé is all you need to gain maximum pleasure, and a whole dessert is often too much for all of us.

Stop wasting your money on cheap pizza, no-name chocolates and mass-produced cakes that fill a boredom or habit hole – be fussy with your food and enjoy the best!

No eating after 8pm

'The earlier you have your breakfast and dinner,
the better it is for your metabolism.'

Long gone are the days when we ate our breakfast at 7am, lunch at noon
and dinner at 6pm sharp. Instead we are lucky to eat breakfast by 9am,
lunch by 2pm and dinner by 9pm. With longer working hours and later
meals, our metabolisms are not so happy. In fact, eating later may be a
strong determinant of weight gain over time.

The human body is programmed according to what is called a circadian
rhythm. This means the hormones that regulate our digestive system
burn our food during the day and store energy at night. The simple life
shift that sees many of us eating our meals later and later, often with our
most energy-dense meal at night, means we are setting ourselves up
for weight gain metabolically. In order to make the most of our natural
metabolism, we need to shift our eating habits forward. The midmorning
hunger people often complain of after an early breakfast is actually a good
thing – it means your body has burnt all the calories from its first meal
and is ready to be fuelled up again.

The first thing we can do to shift things forward is to always eat breakfast
and do so earlier – 9 or 10am is just too late. You have basically missed
2–3 hours of your own metabolic kickstart. Even if you are not hungry

when you first wake, get into the habit of having something small – a single slice of toast with some cheese or baked beans, a protein shake, half a bowl of oats or muesli. Then as you gradually reprogramme your body and eat less at night, you will find you wake up hungrier and you will be well on your way to shifting your total caloric intake forward so you eat less during the second half of the day.

Ideally the body needs 10–12 hours overnight without food to resume its natural digestive balance. This means that for many of us who are not eating dinner until 8pm, and then following that with dessert or treats late into the evening, we're not giving the body enough time without food and are less likely to wake up hungry the next morning.

There are a few solutions to the eating late at night issue, which is relatively common in busy, over-scheduled lives. The first solution is to choose a light meal if you cannot avoid eating after 8pm. As a general rule of thumb, we need just two small bowls full of food at dinnertime, one filled with vegetables or salad and one with a mix of lean protein and carbohydrates. After 8pm you can get away with just a single bowl of food, made up of mostly vegetables or salad. Remember a reduced dinner means you'll need a larger lunch, which should include at least 1 cup of low-GI carbohydrates, 1–2 cups of vegetables or salad and a palm-sized serving of protein.

The second option to shift things forward is to plan to eat your meal at work at 5 or 6pm, so you only need a small top up when you get home later. This is also a good option for those heading to the gym after work.

For those who are particularly strong-minded, developing a personal mantra such as, 'I do not eat after 8pm', can be a powerful way to self-regulate. This can be conducive to weight loss and lead to healthy food rules becoming practised and entrenched.

Finally, avoid high-fat, high-calorie treats late at night. The extra chocolate, ice-cream, biscuits and desserts can easily contain as much as a quarter of an adult's total daily caloric requirement, consumed at a time when far fewer calories are burnt. Eliminating these high-energy treats late at night is often the difference between losing weight and not. If you love nothing more than enjoying a sweet treat after your meal, keep it very small (less than 100 calories) and limit it to specific nights of the week so it's not a daily habit.

LOW-CALORIE DINNER OMELETTE

olive oil cooking spray

1 egg, lightly beaten with
a dash of low-fat milk

½ small courgette, grated

1 tomato, chopped

¼ red pepper, chopped

2 tablespoons grated
low-fat cheddar cheese

Serves 1

1 Place a non-stick frying pan
over a medium heat. Coat pan
with cooking spray, then add
the egg and swirl to coat the
base of the pan.

2 Sprinkle the egg with the
courgette, tomato, pepper
and cheese. Cook for 2 minutes,
or until the egg has set, then
turn the omelette over and
cook the other side. Serve with
a salad.

Be smart when eating out

'For those who eat out regularly, knowing what to order goes a long way to keeping your weight under control.'

We all need to know some simple tricks to master the delicate balance of enjoying our favourite cuisines and restaurants without a complete calorie overload. Unfortunately restaurant meals often mean extra calories thanks to larger portion sizes, the liberal use of oil, butter and sauces as well as numerous courses.

CHOOSE YOUR CUISINES CAREFULLY

While we are blessed with a myriad of options when it comes to eating out, some cuisines offer better choices than others. Indian, Chinese and Thai food in particular tend to be extremely high in fat, due to the use of coconut milk and batters, as well as the large volumes of oil used. When high-fat curries and fried foods are eaten with large amounts of white rice, noodles and bread, it's easy to see how an energy overload can result. Ideally such high-fat cuisines need to be consumed sparingly – just once or twice a month. Be mindful of avoiding the fried choices on the menu. Instead look for plain vegetable curries and stir-fries and try enjoying them with just a small scoop of either rice, noodles or bread.

LOOK FOR THE LIGHT OPTIONS

Lighter options that can be enjoyed more regularly include Japanese and Greek cuisines, as these tend to have a much wider range of menu items that will allow you to make healthier choices. Any sort of raw fish, grilled meat or seafood will be a great choice, especially when teamed with a large portion of vegetables or salad. If you are trying to lose weight, be direct with friends and colleagues when choosing places to dine. Encourage them to visit a restaurant you know has healthy options.

SIZE IS EVERYTHING

One of the biggest issues with eating out is that we tend to eat much more. Few of us really need both a starter as well as a main course and for most of us a starter-sized portion of heavier foods such as pasta or risotto will be more than sufficient. If the portions of pasta, rice or meat are far larger than you need, before you start your meal, visualise how much of the portion you will eat, and then take the excess off your plate and share with your fellow diners. Otherwise learn to be comfortable leaving some food on your plate if you know you are not hungry enough to eat it. If you must have a starter, look for lighter options such as a few grilled seafood pieces, a soup or salad. When it comes to dessert, remember that the most pleasure is gained in the first few mouthfuls, so if you really spot something you love on the menu, share with as many people as possible.

VEGETABLES, VEGETABLES, VEGETABLES

One the biggest issues with meals consumed away from the home is that they rarely contain the amounts of vegetables or salad we need for good health and to help us feel full. Even though they can be expensive when ordered as sides, it's worth ordering extras to help bulk up your meal so you're not tempted by crisps or bread. When eating heavier cuisines such as Indian and Thai, always order an extra vegetable-based dish to reduce the amount of heavy curry and rice that you are likely to eat.

PLAN AHEAD

If you really struggle to limit yourself when you are out, another powerful psychological technique is to plan in advance what will be the best choice for you prior to arriving at the restaurant. This way you won't be overwhelmed with options and make a rash decision. Also when you arrive remember how dreadful you feel when you overeat – this can be a strong deterrent.

WHAT'S THE OCCASION?

Perhaps the most important thing to consider when you're dining out is whether it's a special occasion, or just a regular occurrence. For special occasions enjoyed at amazing restaurants, look for ways to make your meal well-balanced and avoid overeating, but of course take the opportunity to enjoy dessert and other treats you would not usually have. It's the weekly Thai or trip to the local restaurant that does more damage than the one-off celebrations.

Top tips for eating out

1. Never go to a restaurant starving. Have a small snack 1–2 hours before to take the edge off your hunger.
2. Be direct with friends when they're making restaurant choices – remember that both Indian and Thai foods are exceptionally high in fat.
3. If you love eating bread, try doing what the Italians do – take the middle out and just enjoy the crust.
4. Order as much extra salad and as many vegetables as you can to bulk up your plate.
5. Aim to be the last to finish your meal, eating slowly, placing your knife and fork down between each mouthful and chewing everything well.
6. Be mindful that restaurant food is often very salty, so drink at least three glasses of water throughout the meal to help flush away the salt and avoid bloating.
7. If you have overdone things, just make sure your next meal is a light soup or salad to help compensate for the extra calories.
8. Sit with the person who eats the least and likes to eat healthily. You are likely to be influenced by what those around you are ordering so this will help keep you on track.

ENERGY AND FAT CONTENT OF COMMON MEALS OUT			
COMMON CHOICE	**BETTER CHOICE**	**CALORIE SAVING**	**FAT SAVING (g)**
Pad thai	Chicken stir-fry	350	8
Chicken teriyaki	8-pack sushi	300	17
Butter chicken	Tandoori chicken	200	17
Pesto pasta	Spaghetti bolognaise	250	24
3-piece KFC feed	4-piece Nandos pack	600	49
4 slices Meat Lovers pizza	Chicken kebab	400	29
Thai green curry	Pork stir-fry in soy sauce	0	35

Take a meal off

'Restriction rarely works long-term – we need to manage our diet sustainably to control our weight for good.'

Often when we begin a weight-loss programme, we expect to feel deprived, to not be able to eat any of our favourite foods and that the diet will be completely ruined if we eat something that is not on the list. But the truth is that the body actually doesn't respond well to long periods of strict calorie restriction.

Research shows that long periods of time with too few calories can result in the brain releasing neurotransmitters that make you want to eat. It appears that when the body thinks it is starving, it is powerfully driven to seek food, which may be the reason dieters face the intense hunger that makes it so challenging to stay on track after experiencing initial weight loss.

A very easy way to overcome this physiological signalling is to include a meal in your regular diet plan that is 'free', or has more calories than you have been limiting yourself to for the other 6 days of the week. Not only does this give you the freedom to enjoy a meal out or special celebration, but it also gives your body the message that it is not starving and should burn up energy and extra fat as usual – a win–win situation.

Now, please note that the suggestion is to have one meal off – not a whole day, not a four-course buffet, just one meal. This may mean including some carbohydrates at night, it may mean adding in a slice of birthday cake or including a couple of alcoholic drinks on a night out. Overall you should aim for no more than 200–250 extra calories. Follow this meal with some extra movement and then get straight back on to your programme. Such a change will not negatively affect your weight-loss attempt, in fact it may even enhance it.

your BEHAVIOUR

'Only you have control over
what goes into your mouth.'

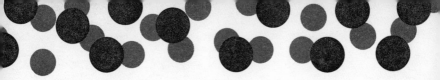

How many times a day does food enter your mouth?

'Once you count the snacks, treats, meals and drinks – many of us are eating 20–30 times a day.'

For one day I want you to keep a record of the number of times any sort of food enters your mouth. Not just your meals, but all the coffees and tea with milk or sugar, snacks, leftovers and treats that slip in over the day. Many of my clients were astounded to find after keeping this record that food was entering their mouths as many as 20–30 times each day, when the number should be more like 6–7 times at most.

The body is programmed to eat a meal and then nothing for at least 2–3 hours. Constant nibbling between meals and snacks disrupts the natural digestive process. When we eat, insulin is secreted to take glucose to the muscles. Insulin is a fat-storing hormone, so every time you eat something, no matter how small, insulin will be secreted, and the more insulin, the more fat storage occurs over time.

Aim to eat only every 2–3 hours with nothing except water or herbal tea in between. This will allow your digestive hormones to function efficiently and help you experience your natural hunger and satiety signals – the best guides when it comes to when and how much you should eat.

Know your eating style

'Some of us binge, others restrict, others need to try everything. Identifying your eating pattern will help you get your weight under control for good.'

Everyone has a different eating style depending on food preferences, what we're taught as children and who we spend our time with, but does your eating style prevent weight loss? Once your pattern has been identified, you can generally manage it with a few basic behavioural strategies.

RESTRICTED EATING

Restrictive eaters base their food choices on what they think they should eat as opposed to what they feel like eating. They tend to have strict food rules but can be prone to overeating when one of these rules is broken. Restrictive eaters are often on a diet, may avoid social situations for fear of not having access to the food they think they should be eating and spend far too much time calculating the fat and calorie content of their diets.

A good starting point is to ask yourself, 'What do I really feel like eating?' Try to remove the cognitive programming entrenched in your mind that tells you certain foods are bad. Once you start challenging these beliefs and eating foods you normally avoid, you will not feel out of control if you do try a dessert or eat a controlled portion of carbohydrates at dinner. Always remember that there are no strict rules about what we should and shouldn't eat – there are balanced meals with everyday foods, and other foods that we eat sometimes in controlled amounts.

EMOTIONAL EATING

Some of us eat less when we are sad, stressed or lonely while some of us eat more. Emotional eating is frequently reported as a behavioural side effect of emotional distress, and if not identified and managed early can result in extra body weight courtesy of chocolates, ice-creams and biscuits – the most common foods sought out by emotional eaters.

The first thing to do is identify the emotional triggers that lead you to eat high-calorie food. Then you can practise having a 'time out' in between the trigger and the eating – try calling a friend, getting out of the house or office (a change in environment works very effectively) or writing down the pros and cons of eating your desired treat. This breathing space makes it much easier to think rationally about eating rather than rushing to the fridge and downing a tub of ice-cream. If you are prone to emotional overeating, never keep your comfort foods in the house. Having to go out to buy them puts time in between the crisis point and when the food is available, which will help you to make a rational decision not to binge.

THE SERIAL DIETER

You name it, the serial dieter has tried it! Low-carb, high-protein, cabbage only – but the serial dieter never seems to lose weight. Too much energy is spent on fad diets instead of developing long-term healthy eating behaviour.

If you are a serial dieter, think about all the precious time and energy (not to mention money) you have wasted on these programmes for no outcome. In fact, serial dieting tends to have a negative impact on metabolic rate long-term and can be particularly limiting psychologically if each diet has resulted in failure. If you are serious about getting healthy, book yourself into a dietitian and get a balanced, personalised food plan to deal with your weight issues once and for all.

THE EVENING BINGER

Evening bingers eat next to nothing all day, arrive home famished and eat everything in sight. Consuming a disproportionate number of calories during the second half of the day means low energy levels in the morning and long-term weight gain, as high-calorie foods are often chosen at this time, when your body has switched from fat-burning to fat-storage mode.

If you are a night binger, you need to get organised and support your metabolism rather than sabotage it. Practise planning ahead each day so you have all the food supplies you need for at least three meals each day. Try having a protein-rich snack such as a cereal bar, milk-based drink or protein bar on the way home from work so you don't walk in the door ravenous. Like emotional eaters, you may find it helps to not keep 'easy to eat' snacks such as biscuits, dips, chocolates and potato crisps at home as they are too easy to overeat when you're starving.

THE HEALTH FANATIC

Health fanatics may look fabulous from a distance but a closer look can reveal dry skin, fatigue and low moods as the obsession with all things natural and healthy has resulted in a life without much pleasure. While eating nutritionally balanced food should be a goal for all of us, taking it to an extreme where you won't eat out or eat any type of food unless it is organic, natural and unprocessed can become mentally draining and lead to obsession.

If you cannot remember the last time you ate out or even enjoyed your food, you need to loosen the food rules a little. There is nothing wrong with healthy eating but if it's limiting you socially, there is a problem. To break free of this health obsession, think about what foods you really enjoy eating and make sure you have those included in your meal plan. Practise eating out at new places and making decisions on regular menu items. And most importantly, remember that food is meant to nourish your body and eating is meant to be a pleasurable experience. If you do not find this is the case, you may need to speak to a professional on issues relating to control in your life.

Food habits
that make you fat

*'You have the power and the opportunity
to change your habits.'*

It is not the one-off trip to your favourite fast-food shop or bakery that
results in you carrying extra weight – it's the extra calories that slip in
on a daily basis because of the poor food habits you've developed over
time. The extra coffee at work, eating the kids' leftovers or enjoying a
high-calorie treat every night after dinner … The first step towards kicking
bad food habits is to identify them. When do you notice yourself eating
something not because you are hungry but because it is there? When do
you look forward to a food reward throughout the day? Here are some of
the most common poor food habits.

EATING IN THE CAR
Eating in the car starts when we're running late, then it becomes
something we do every day to save time and before you know it, you
find yourself always looking for food when you're behind the wheel.

The link between driving and food means you are more likely to look
for a service station to purchase unhealthy snacks and coffees every time
you're driving for extended periods. Make a commitment to not eat in the

car at all and instead always keep your water bottle and some mints with you for when you need something in your mouth but know you don't need the calories.

EATING IN FRONT OF THE TV

Eating in front of the TV is a terrible habit of modern life. We get home late and reward ourselves with a quick meal in front of our favourite sitcom or DVD. The issue with this is that we're not concentrating on how much we're eating and hence are likely to overeat.

Make a commitment to only eat food sitting down at the table – no excuses. Studies have shown that individuals eat more calories throughout the course of the day when they have eaten meals in front of the TV. Not paying attention to what you're eating affects your ability to self-monitor. If you must, limit it to just once a week, on a Sunday for example, so you are at lower risk of the habit developing again when you're tired. Keep your eating area, such as the kitchen or dining table, clear so it's easy to sit and eat a meal there, and create a nice environment with a candle or music so that you link dinner to feeling relaxed and comfortable, especially if you have small children.

SOMETHING SWEET AT 3PM

Remember that a strong craving for intense flavour, whether it be sweet or savoury, generally means that your meal beforehand did not contain enough bulky salad vegetables and/or protein. While eating at 3pm can become a habit, if there's an underlying physiological reason why you're looking for these flavours at certain times, at some point you need to work out why so you can manage it and ideally prevent the craving.

First check your lunch to make sure that you've included both a good source of protein and salad or vegetables. If you still crave something sweet at 3pm, try not to wait until the craving is extreme before you eat. Have something savoury first and notice how this takes away your craving for sugar rather than feeding it. Crackers with low-fat cheese or cream cheese are a good choice. Then if you also eat something small and sweet such as a single low-fat cookie, some fresh fruit or a portion-controlled chocolate, you will have also had the savoury food to help regulate your blood glucose levels for the rest of the afternoon.

GORGING BEFORE DINNER

It's common to have an extreme urge to eat when you get home from work as it's been several hours since lunch. The key is to prevent this intense hunger so you're more in control when making your food choice.

The easiest strategy to prevent late-afternoon hunger is to get into a habit of grabbing an apple or carrot to eat on the way home from work. This way you've eaten something healthy and taken the edge off your hunger, so you're less likely to overdo it and spoil your dinner.

EATING THE KIDS' LEFTOVERS

This is an easy trap for parents to fall into, generally because they prioritise the kids' needs over their own, and because it's easy to pick at food in front of you.

First of all, if you routinely have leftovers from your kids' meals, you are preparing too much food. Get used to putting leftovers in containers immediately to reserve for later so that you're not tempted. Most importantly, prioritise your own food needs so you don't get over-hungry. Remember, parents who look after themselves are in a better place mentally and physically to care for their children.

Are your friends making you fat?

'We become like the people we spend our time with.'

Yes, sad but true. If your friends are lean, fit and healthy you are significantly more likely to be so. If, on the other hand, your friends could all lose a bit of weight and you're more likely to catch up over a coffee and cake as opposed to a run and vegetable juice, things are not looking great.

Why does this happen? For all our education and self-awareness, we all simply want to be like everyone else. In groups of people, whether it's at work, within a family or in a partnership, it's far easier to conform than it is to change the norm. This is why corporate weight-loss challenges work in the short-term – everyone is involved in the programme, which creates group energy that everyone wants to be a part of. But unless such changes become the norm within the organisation, things will peter out once the programme is over.

Now this doesn't mean you have to go and get rid of all your friends. Simply being more aware of the powerful influence friends and acquaintances can have over your daily food and activity decisions is all you need to instigate changes. If you always meet friends over a meal or snack, suggest that exercise also becomes part of it. Seek out those people in your world who are also committed to health and fitness and use their energy to support you in initiating and making changes. In extreme cases where too much focus is put on food and eating, or if you find that your friends are actually sabotaging your diet efforts, you may need to draw the inappropriate behaviour to their attention. Honestly and openly state your plans to lose weight or to eat better, and request their support to help you achieve this goal. In more cases than not you will find that your friends are actually keen to eat better and lose a bit around the middle too. You may just need to be the strong influencer to get things moving.

Seeking out the company of other fit and healthy people can be a very powerful way to move towards a life of health and fitness. Joining running, walking or cycling clubs, triathlon groups, mums' groups or fitness and yoga groups are all ways to meet like-minded people and start to incorporate health and fitness into your life.

Are your hormones making you fat?

'Hormones play havoc with our lives when we're teenagers and havoc with our weight when we're adults.'

For many years, scientists, nutritionists and numerous other weight-loss professionals have preached that weight loss comes down to a very simple equation – calories in versus calories out. While this principle is true to a certain extent, it is a little too simplistic. There are a number of hormonal shifts that can occur to alter this relationship. One such diagnosis is insulin resistance, the clinical condition that precedes type 2 diabetes. Individuals with insulin resistance will struggle to lose weight via traditional weight-loss methods simply because their body is not burning fuel the way it should be.

As discussed earlier, insulin is a hormone secreted by the pancreas and used to digest carbohydrates. When carbohydrate-rich foods are consumed, insulin is secreted by the pancreas to take glucose from the bloodstream to the muscles for energy. For a number of reasons, over time, insulin may fail to work as well as it should. Weight gain, where fat is clogging the cells, is such a reason, as is a lack of physical activity. Your genetics can also predispose you to insulin resistance and type 2 diabetes. Another significant contributing factor to insulin resistance is the highly processed nature of our daily carb choices including breads, breakfast cereals and snack foods, which require much higher amounts of insulin than less-processed low-GI carbs.

Resistance to insulin builds up over time, with the body gradually producing more and more insulin to get glucose out of the blood and into the body's cells for energy. As insulin is also a fat-storing hormone, the more of it that's circulating in the body, the harder it becomes to actually burn body fat. High levels of insulin can also make you feel tired and bloated and crave sugar, as the body is not getting the fuel it needs to the cells as efficiently as it should be. Individuals with insulin resistance also tend to have distinct abdominal fat deposits and carry much of their weight around their belly.

Once diagnosed by a physician or endocrinologist, insulin resistance can be managed. Tight management can actually prevent the development of type 2 diabetes. While some cases will warrant medication, the diet and exercise prescription does not change. Individuals with insulin resistance need a reduced-carb, increased-protein diet developed by a specialist dietitian, as well as a highly specific training programme that integrates high-intensity cardio sessions in conjunction with a light resistance-training programme. Individuals with insulin resistance need to learn to become extremely fussy with their choice of carbs. High-GI carbs, including juice, white bread and refined cereals, need to be completely eliminated from the diet for the best weight-loss outcomes long-term.

Signs that you may have a degree of insulin resistance that may be worth investigating include an inability to lose weight despite a healthy diet and exercise routine, distinct abdominal fat, feeling unusually fatigued, bloating and craving sugar regularly. Identifying insulin resistance early and committing to a 6–12 month diet and exercise intervention may help you avoid getting diabetes.

So if you are a veteran of the weight-loss industry and cannot seem to lose weight no matter which diet you try, it may be time for a trip to your doctor for a glucose-tolerance test (with insulin levels) to be performed after you have eaten a high-carb diet for 3 days. The test will check how your hormones are responding to sugar when it's present in your blood. High insulin levels on this test indicate that your hormones are working too hard to maintain an optimal blood glucose level, which will fast track you to type 2 diabetes if not managed.

Reset your hunger switch

'When was the last time you felt really, really hungry?'

Although hunger is the primary physiological cue to tell us that we need more food, very few of us eat solely according to our hunger signals. We eat because food is in front of us, because it is a meal or snack time, because we're bored or because we're scared that we might get hungry later.

Failing to eat according to hunger over long periods of time means that we are at risk of constantly overeating, and hence making our food choices externally rather than internally driven. This means we eat more and more, and programme our belly and head into thinking we need more food than we actually do. If you cannot remember the last time you actually felt really hungry, it's time to reset your hunger. Ideally we need to feel hungry every 2–3 hours. Hunger is a sign that you're burning your food well. It is a sign that your metabolism is working optimally.

Often people who eat too much at night don't wake up hungry and then skip breakfast. Such a behavioural pattern is not only shifting your caloric intake towards the second half of the day, but means that you're skipping your early morning hunger signal. Some claim they don't eat breakfast because it actually makes them hungrier throughout the morning. But such regular hunger is a good thing, it's a sign a dormant metabolism is kicking in.

To reset your hunger switch, try having a very light meal at 5 or 6pm for your dinner. Good options include a vegetable soup (see recipe on the following page) or some sushi. Then wait at least 12–14 hours until you eat a large breakfast of eggs on toast or muesli the next morning. Not only should you be hungry for this meal, but you should be satisfied until midmorning when you need to eat something that will again fill you for 2–3 hours.

If you actually feel nauseous in the mornings and really cannot tolerate anything, start reintroducing breakfast slowly. Remember that your body has not been used to eating so early for some time so it will take time to reprogramme it. Start with a small snack first thing such as a couple of plain crackers. Over time you will notice your morning appetite improves as long as you keep your evening meal light and enjoy it by 8pm.

PUMPKIN & CARROT SOUP

4 large carrots, diced

½ pumpkin, peeled and diced

dill sprigs to serve

shaved parmesan to serve

1 Place the carrot and pumpkin in a large saucepan and cover with water. Bring to the boil, reduce the heat to a simmer and cook until the vegetables are soft.

2 Allow the soup to cool slightly, then purée using a hand-held blender, or in batches in a food processor or blender.

3 Return the soup to the pan and season to taste with rock salt or sea salt. Gently reheat until warmed through. Serve garnished with dill and parmesan.

Serves 4–6

Change your food routine

'If you've eaten the same breakfast, lunch and snacks for the past 5 years and your body's not changing, it may be time to mix things up.'

The body likes things to be stable, including your weight. If you have eaten the same thing for the past 5 years, it is likely your body hasn't had to work hard to digest your food for some time. The best thing you can do to kick start it is to change things around and get it working a little harder. So, if you always eat cereal and fruit for breakfast, swap to eggs and toast for a while. If you usually enjoy a big breakfast with no snacks, swap to a small breakfast and add in a midmorning snack instead. If you have three square meals, swap to six small ones.

Research has shown that dieters who alter their daily food intake pattern to consume 50 per cent of their total daily calories at breakfast lost significantly more body fat on a weight-loss diet than individuals who continued eating their regular calorie profile. Weight-loss diets have also shown that individuals are more likely to reach their goal weight if they start with a stricter regime compared to a more gradual reduction in calories.

Another slightly more prescriptive dietary approach is to aggressively cycle the number of calories that you eat each day. Known as the 'alternate day' approach, this programme suggests dieters alternate between high or regular calorie-intake days (1500–2000 calories) and light calorie-intake days (as few as 800–1000 calories) for short periods of time. With such radical differences in caloric intake, the metabolism is constantly challenged, which can be all that's needed to shift dieters from a plateau or get their hunger and fullness signals firing again. While such an approach may seem extreme, if done properly for short periods of time there are no detrimental side effects. Try alternating 2–3 days of regular eating with a day of very low calorie eating and see if your own hunger signals get a move along.

SAMPLE CALORIE-CYCLE MEAL PLANS		
MEAL	800 CALORIE PROGRAMME	1500 CALORIE PROGRAMME
Breakfast	Protein shake	1 egg + 1 toast + 1 fruit
Midmorning	Berries	Cheese and crackers + low-fat coffee
Lunch	Tuna salad	Tuna salad sandwich
Midafternoon	10 walnuts + apple	Cereal bar + fruit
Dinner	50g meat + vegetables	150g meat + vegetables

Mindless munching

'When we eat mindfully, we eat less and enjoy our food more. Eat slowly, chew your food, savour.'

Since the term 'mindless eating' was explored in depth by eating-behaviour researcher Brian Wansink, more attention has been paid to not only what we eat but the way we do it. Mindless eating occurs when we're not paying attention – a handful of jelly beans, a couple of bites of the kids' leftovers, the pre-dinner snack of cheese and crackers while you chop the vegetables. When we're not paying attention to what goes in our mouths, we're likely to eat far more than we need, to not register that we've eaten it and to fail to compensate at our next meal. Being more mindful about the way we eat is crucial in avoiding extra calories slipping into our day, resulting in extra weight gain long-term.

Mindless eating occurs when you're distracted or doing something else. Eating when driving, watching TV or preparing dinner, for example. It can easily become a habit when you naturally link a certain situation to eating – grabbing a chocolate bar when filling the car with petrol or saying yes to coffee and cake by default when meeting friends.

To gain control of this type of mindless eating, keep a record of the times food is entering your mouth and then ask yourself, 'Am I hungry, or is eating that food at that time just a bad habit?' Once you recognise when you're eating out of habit, the easier it will be to stop yourself.

The next step in controlling mindless eating is to limit the amount of food you have around you. Rid your home, office and social environments of as much visible food stimulus as you can. It is time to clear the desk or bench of snacks, the office kitchen of the visible biscuit jar and the car of hidden snacks. Not having food in front of you all the time will make you less likely to think about it outside of meal times. You will start eating out of hunger, rather than in response to visual stimulus.

Mindless eating also occurs when we eat too quickly. Too often we find ourselves rushing to get a meal down so we can move on to our next task. It takes the stomach at least 20 minutes to register that it's had enough food, which is often a few hundred calories after we put the fork down. Recent research has found that diners who were told to chew each mouthful of food at least 20 times, in addition to placing their knife and fork down in between mouthfuls, consumed 20 per cent fewer calories during a meal than those given no such instructions.

Simply being more aware of the need to slow down will naturally see you take more time with each mouthful and each meal. Chew each mouthful carefully and practise placing your knife and fork down in between each mouthful. Aim to always be the last to finish your meal and take a sip of water in between mouthfuls. Cutting your food into smaller pieces also helps to draw the meal out. Finally, always allow a decent amount of time to pass between courses. You'll find you can only eat a couple of mouthfuls of a dessert when you have really let your food settle, as opposed to the whole helping if you eat it immediately after your meal.

Eating mindfully requires you to concentrate on your food. This means savouring each mouthful, chewing it properly and focusing solely on the eating experience. Being more aware of how much you've eaten will put you in a better position to regulate your energy intake.

Mindless eating traps to avoid

- In the car
- In front of the TV
- In front of the computer
- While reading
- At the desk
- At the kitchen bench
- When preparing dinner

Develop your self-regulation skills

'In a world of food opportunities, self-regulation is what differentiates those who control their weight from those who don't.'

You know how there are the people who can eat half a chocolate bar and leave the rest, or decline offers of dessert no matter how appealing it looks? Or who can skip dinner when they've eaten too much at lunch? Such people have extremely good self-regulatory skills, which will serve them well in many facets of their life, including weight control.

Self-regulation refers to the way in which an individual is able to use self-monitoring and feedback to plan, guide and maintain changes in behaviour to successfully reach their goals. Some aspects of self-regulation are likely to be innate, governed by such physiological signals as hunger and satiety while others are taught to us by parents and other social influencers.

The most primitive of food-related self-regulatory variables – hunger and satiety – are innate. Babies, for example, are very good at telling their mothers when they are hungry and when they have had enough. But the rapidly growing rate of obesity suggests that these cues are easily overridden. We all know it's easy to overeat, yet not so easy to skip a meal.

It's easy to allow one drink to turn into four, or one row of chocolate to become an entire block. Such programmed behaviour is easy to repeat time and time again when it is all we have ever known. In such instances, food is not being consumed because of taste or desire but rather as instant reward and part of a learnt habit.

We each have a different required level of self-regulation that will allow us to control our food intake and our weight. For example, some of us will self-regulate by eating well during the week while relaxing things a little at weekends, while others will judge the degree of self-regulation required by keeping an eye on the scales or belt notches to determine when things appear to be creeping up.

If you know that you lack self-regulatory skills, the first step towards improving them is to determine where they are most lacking. Is it when you drink alcohol? When you are alone at home or when you are eating with friends? Once you are more aware of where your self-regulation abilities are lacking (exercise, food behaviours or both), you are in a position to improve your skills – to be able to clearly state that you will only be having two drinks or that you will skip the chips with your meal. Once you have one or two self-regulatory strategies you will be in a much better position to start to govern the rules around these cues. As is the case with any new habit, practice will be required in order for these skills to translate into normal behaviour. The good news is that 3 months after a new behaviour is adopted, you will find that you no longer need to think about it – the healthy decision will come naturally.

Top 10 tips for self-regulation

1   Before you enter a shop, decide whether or not you will be purchasing food.

2   Avoid service station money-making schemes offering you '2-for-1' on high-fat, high-calorie foods such as chocolate bars. Try not to look at the food items around the counter at all – out of sight, out of mind.

3   If you are hungry, look for protein bars, cereal bars and low-fat milk drinks, or purchase gum or mints instead of food.

4   Have clear rules about the foods you will eat at certain times – for example, only eat crisps on weekends.

5   Always keep a protein-rich snack with you in your bag or car to avoid getting over hungry.

6   Give yourself just one occasion each week to eat high-calorie foods such as fast food, biscuits, cakes and chocolates.

7   When enjoying high-calorie food such as fried food or pizza, make a mental decision on how much you will allow yourself to enjoy before you start eating.

8   Only serve the quantity of food you know you should be having, even if you feel hungry.

9   Always wait at least 20 minutes before allowing yourself second helpings or dessert.

10   Start eating less by aiming to always leave at least some of your meal on your plate without feeling the need to finish it.

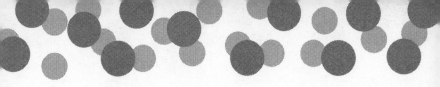

Managing cravings

'You never need to be a victim to your cravings.'

Many people are victims of their food cravings. They fight the desire for salty, sweet or fatty foods until they can no longer manage the mental battle and completely give in, generally eating much more than they need to feel satisfied.

Food cravings actually give us valuable information about what is going on in our bodies. For example, craving sweet foods late in the afternoon generally means that you haven't eaten enough protein and/or salad with your lunch and need to refuel. A craving can also be the result of programming the body to look for certain taste sensations at certain times of day. If you always eat a biscuit with your morning coffee, your brain is going to be looking for a biscuit every day at 10am until you break the association.

Physiological cravings are completely within your control. Significant drops in blood glucose levels (which occur when uneven amounts of carbohydrates are consumed throughout the day) are the most common reason we crave sugar. If you go without carbs or choose the wrong types, you leave yourself vulnerable to extreme sugar highs and lows. Simply aim to eat a slowly digested, low-GI carb every 3–4 hours, even in very small amounts, to help support optimal blood glucose regulation and prevent sugar cravings.

Behavioural cravings can easily be broken by undoing the food link to certain times of day, particularly to extremely sweet and/or salty foods. Breaking the link by going cold turkey on the food you crave is ideal, but a more gentle craving management plan is to first just delay the craving. Rather than instantly eating the food you crave, try and have at least 10 minutes doing something else. You'll be surprised how many times you can eliminate this need for sugar or fat by simply slowing down the eating process and reconsidering. A recent study found that a significant number of participants lost their craving for chocolate when they had to go for a walk before they were allowed to indulge the craving.

Secondly, never feed a craving with more of the same type of food. Remember that foods typically craved often have a rich taste and mouth feel. Giving the body more of this intense flavour and texture is only likely to make the craving worse in future.

Next, you need to change the taste in your mouth. Green tea or iced water with a lemon slice are great ways to kill a craving for sugar, as are sugar-free gum and mints. Brushing your teeth is also a proven technique to quell cravings.

Top tips to manage cravings

1 Consider why you may be craving certain tastes and what you really need to eat to satisfy yourself. Did you eat enough protein at lunch or have you drunk enough water?

2 When a craving hits, ask yourself if it's really hunger you're feeling or are you simply tired or bored and filling that need with unnecessary calories?

3 If you do eat that food, will you be able to stop?

4 Instead of eating junk food when you have a craving, eat something healthy instead so you feel full and satisfied.

5 Drink some green tea or brush your teeth to help you neutralise your palate.

Learn to stop overeating

*'Just as you have taught yourself to overeat,
you can teach yourself not to.'*

We all eat high-calorie, high-fat foods from time to time and have
periods where we overeat, whether due to boredom, celebration,
comfort or not having the ability to clearly identify hunger. If indulgence
happens occasionally at celebrations and parties it's not such an issue.
For those of us who find ourselves overeating regularly and gaining
weight as a result, it's time to take a closer look at why the overeating
is occurring.

Overeating is extremely easy because the body lets it happen. If fullness
was anywhere near as strong a sensation as hunger, few of us would have
issues regulating the volume of food we eat. If it's been some time since
you have managed to stop eating at the right time, it's time to get back in
touch with your body's natural appetite signals. Signs that you may be
overdoing it on a regular basis include not feeling hungry, being able to
eat much larger volumes of food than you had previously and, of course,
the clothes getting tighter.

Try serving yourself much smaller portions, even half of your regular
meal if you have to, and eat as slowly as possible. Try ending the meal
a mouthful or so before you usually would to remind yourself of what
feeling comfortably full feels like. Such a process will take time – weeks or

even months – but it's important to work through it to remind yourself of the body's natural hunger and satiety signals.

The most important thing to do if you or other family members are prone to overeating is to limit the type and volume of food that is kept in the home. Forget the idea of having a chocolate stash in your desk that you'll only raid in emergencies or keeping a packet of biscuits in the cupboard that you'll only open if guests visit, because if it's there you will eat it.

Another strategy to implement as you seek to gain control is to compensate when you do overindulge. Learning to balance indulgences rather than trying to avoid them altogether is the key to weight control success. This simply means that if you've overdone it for a meal, make sure you cut back on the next. Longer periods of indulgence in turn need longer periods of compensation. A week of holiday eating equals a week of eating lightly.

The best light options to balance your diet during these periods of lighter eating include vegetable-based juice, broth-style soups, meal-replacement shakes and salads. The secret to compensating well is to not let yourself starve. As soon as you are starving (either psychologically with small volumes of food or literally with inadequate nutrition), the more difficult it will be to stay on track with your lighter diet. Instead, leave your diet with the same volume of food but with fewer calories.

Top 10 tips to avoid overeating

1   Plan your meals and snacks so you don't get too hungry and prone to overeating.
2   Avoid buffets.
3   Put leftovers away before you sit down to eat your meal.
4   Eat lightly during the day if you're going out for dinner.
5   End your meal with something small and sweet.
6   Go for a walk after meals to get out of the kitchen.
7   Don't over shop. Buy only what you need each week.
8   Have a snack before you attend social occasions where food will be served.
9   Quantify your hunger and aim to only eat when you are at 8–9 out of 10.
10 Chew gum or brush your teeth after meals.

Think thin

'Thin people always eat less and exercise more than you do.'

Over the past 10 years a number of studies have been published detailing the behaviour of individuals who not only manage to lose relatively large amounts of weight but who manage to keep it off. It's a very simple mix of behaviours repeated each day that allows individuals to live a lifestyle they enjoy while still controlling their weight.

KEEP MOVING

Thin people move their bodies for an hour each day. Note this does not say, 'flog their bodies for an hour each day' or 'see a personal trainer three times a week' – just move. Learn to incorporate incidental exercise into each day, no matter how small; walking to and from the station, taking the stairs, getting off the bus a stop early, not taking the lift, picking up the kids from school on foot – whatever takes your fancy.

NIP IT IN THE BUD

Thin people monitor their weight closely – no waiting until they've gained three sizes before they take drastic diet action. Weigh yourself once a week to make sure you're not creeping up and, if you have, cut back then and there before the problem becomes unmanageable.

STAY ON TRACK

Thin people don't change their diet regime. It doesn't matter if it's the Christmas season, a trip away, winter – thin people stick to a basic diet regime that works for them. Sure, they may take a break in order to enjoy a special meal but they are back on track the very next day.

NO FAD DIETING

Thin people follow a basic diet containing few processed foods – not low-carb or high-protein, not counting calories or fats, simply avoiding processed foods such as cakes, biscuits, fried foods and pastries, and eating plenty of fresh fruit and vegetables as a way of life.

NEVER SKIP BREAKFAST

Thin people always eat breakfast – every day, no exceptions. This keeps their metabolism functioning at the optimal level – burning energy at the time of day they need it most, which is better for their bodies long-term.

HAVE BACK-UP

Thin people have a great support crew – friends, family and work colleagues who directly or indirectly support their weight-control regimes. Whether by not sabotaging their routine, motivating them to be more active or providing emotional support when it's needed, those people around them help keep their diet and exercise regimes on track.

DO IT FOR YOURSELF

Thin people stay thin because they want to – they don't lose weight to fit into a dress on Saturday night or to look good for their 10-year high school reunion. Thin people look after their body and their weight because they know they will look, feel and function better if they do. They value themselves and know that their health and fitness has to come first if they are to be at their best. This keeps them on track and committed.

KNOW WHAT WORKS FOR YOU

Thin people know what they need to do to control their weight – they know how much they can eat and they know how much training they need to do to keep their weight under control no matter what circumstance they find themselves in. At some point they've taken the time and energy required to develop a diet and exercise regime that works for them so they are able to stick it.

NO EXCUSES

Thin people take responsibility and don't blame others for skipping training sessions or eating too much. They accept that only they have the power to maintain their regime and healthy weight as a result.

DON'T SACRIFICE YOUR REGIME TO STRESS

Thin people don't turn to food when stressed or emotional. They find other ways to soothe and distract themselves and don't use stress as an excuse to skip training sessions.

Expect a plateau

'Plateaus are part of the weight-loss process and should be expected.'

A common weight-loss scenario is to have an initial successful weight loss of 6–11lb after some diet modification, then nothing. Nothing happens on the scales for a couple of weeks and sometimes your weight may even increase by a pound or so. Why does this happen and how can you move yourself off the dreaded weight-loss plateau?

Weight-loss plateaus occur for a very simple reason. The human body likes to be stable and doesn't like losing weight. Once it has lost weight it works better, we know this, but the body perceives weight loss as a negative energy state and will do everything it can to halt this loss. If the body thinks it is receiving too few calories or if weight has been lost rapidly, the metabolism may in fact be slowed in order to conserve energy. This is the most common reason weight loss slows down when food intake has been reduced for extended periods of time.

There are several strategies that can be implemented to move you off a weight-loss plateau. Ironically, in many cases you may have to eat a little more. Following a very low-calorie or low-carbohydrate food plan for extended periods of time may have pushed the metabolism to breaking point. So to kickstart things, try increasing your calories slightly – just 100–200 extra each day – by increasing the size of your breakfast or lunch while still keeping your energy intake low during the second half of the day. Another option is to keep your diet strict during the first half of the week before relaxing a little over the weekend and enjoying larger meals or the alcohol or dessert you've been skipping.

Other tricks to try include eating breakfast earlier, as well as alternating the size of your breakfast, aiming to be hungry by midmorning. Not experiencing hunger may mean that your meals are being consumed too late in the day or are too large. Your breakfast should keep you full for 2–3 hours. If you are hungry after an hour, your breakfast does not have the right balance of protein and carbs. Try changing your breakfast choice to be hungry for a light snack midmorning. This means your body is burning its food well and your metabolism is firing up.

Finally, just as importantly as altering your food volumes, check your training intensity. Training before breakfast can be a great way to get the metabolism moving. The same goes for changing the type and duration of your regular training. Remember, keeping your body guessing is the answer to both getting off a weight-loss plateau and kick-starting your metabolic rate.

your **BODY**

'The sooner you accept that you need to move your body every day, the sooner you'll be able to focus your energy on finding a training plan that works for you.'

Start small

*'There's no point starting an ambitious gym routine
and only getting through one week – build your training
regime gradually.'*

If you want to enjoy your favourite foods while controlling your weight,
you need to exercise regularly. We know that exercise is good for us for a
myriad of reasons but we also know that busy lifestyles may not always be
conducive to regular workouts, particularly if exercise has never been
a priority in your life.

The beautiful thing about exercise is that if done the right way, at the right
time, it teaches your body to burn food better. The better your body is
able to burn food, the more food you will be able to eat. For the majority
of us who really like to eat, this can only be a good thing. But if exercise
isn't done regularly or effectively, it may leave you prone to hunger and
over-compensation, and in exactly the same place weight-wise.

The rule of thumb for those beginning to incorporate regular exercise into
their lives is to start gently. Rather than committing to five or six sessions
a week right away, only to give up completely a week or two later because
it's too hard, start with one session each week. The key to success with any
new routine is to ensure you choose an activity that you like and is easy
for you to do, and schedule it for a day and time when few distractions
will come up. As soon as a commitment becomes complex – involving

commutes, traffic, children, work finishing on time or an activity you are not that keen on, the chances that you will get there decrease significantly.

The easiest option by far is to walk for just 20–30 minutes first thing in the morning. A small time commitment is less likely to be overwhelming, you can get it out of the way before you start your day and no matter what fitness level you are at, you can manage it. Remember that a walk you do once a week, every week for the rest of your life is going to be much better than a gym class you do for 2 weeks and never again. Start small and build – the easier it fits into your already chaotic schedule, the better.

Top 10 easy ways to move more

1. Get off the bus or the train a stop earlier.
2. Park as far away from your destination as you can.
3. Use the bathroom on a different level in the office.
4. Always take the stairs.
5. If there are no stairs, walk up escalators.
6. Get out and run errands every lunchtime.
7. Stand up at least every hour at work.
8. If you have a question for someone in the office, go and ask them in person rather than sending an email.
9. Always volunteer to pick up the coffees.
10. Walk after dinner.

Measure your body

'Measurements tell us more about the health of our body than our weight ever will.'

Are you terrified of the scales? Would you rather die than have to get on the scales in front of other people? It is safe to say, you are not alone. Scale phobias have often been developed at a young age stemming from uncomfortable memories of a doctor's appointment or gym class when our weight was exposed for all to see, and of course it was a weight that was much higher than we would have liked.

While body weight can be used as a rough marker of health and fitness, for anyone who trains regularly, body composition is a much more insightful marker of health and a more accurate measure of body fat. If you are 14st and should be 11st, there is no doubt that you want to see reductions on the scales over time. But if you are 10st and want to be 9.5st, and your body weight doesn't change but your measurements decrease significantly, it is still an excellent weight-loss outcome. This means you're losing body fat while maintaining muscle mass.

Solely judging your weight loss outcome on shifting scale readings, especially when we're dealing with relatively small amounts of body weight, is almost certainly setting yourself up to fail. You need to take body measurements as well as weight to really monitor how your body is changing. For men, a simple waist measurement is all you need, while women can benefit from a waist, hip, bust and bottom measurement. Never weigh or measure yourself more than once each week, as body weight and size can differ by as much as 2–4.5lb over the course of the day. Always take your measurements first thing in the morning and remember that if you have a salty meal the night before you take the measurements, your weight may be up as much as 2–4.5lb thanks to the fluid retention your body encourages to balance out the extra salt.

For the scale addicts out there who weigh themselves multiple times per week, or even per day, this behaviour is likely to be keeping weight on. Psychologically, not seeing positive progress can often reinforce the desire to go off track with the mentality, 'well it's not working anyway'. People with this level of weight-loss obsession need to be banned from the scales for at least a month and then limited to weighing and measuring at most once each week to regain some perspective. Your focus should be on your general health and fitness, not a number.

Get a pedometer

'It's not just the time you spend on the treadmill, but what you do in between.'

Do you know how many steps you walk each day? Not on the treadmill or with your running group, but as part of your daily routine? If you have no idea, it is time to invest in a wonderful little gadget called a pedometer.

An adult needs to take at least 10,000 steps a day just to maintain their weight. If you want to actually lose weight, you need to bump that number right up to 12,000–20,000. To give you some idea of the distance and time you have to travel to clock up these numbers, you are looking at about an hour for every 7500–10,000 steps. The average office worker who drives to and from work will be lucky to manage 2000 steps each day. No wonder many of us feel tired, bloated and just uncomfortable as we sit and constrict our digestive organs.

A great lifestyle habit you can get into is to go for a 20–30-minute walk after dinner, rather than sitting down, leaving your full belly compacted, bloated and uncomfortable. What do you usually do after your evening meal? Sit on the couch and watch TV? Clean up the kitchen? Collapse into bed? Eat chocolate with a cup of tea? An evening walk not only creates a fantastic time window for families to communicate without the distractions of TV and computers but it also has a great effect on gut comfort and digestion. Your food will have a chance to settle and move through the digestive tract and leave you feeling lighter and more likely to sleep better as a result.

It's routine that sees us develop and maintain healthy lifestyles. Exercising needs to become the same as brushing our teeth before we get into bed or clearing the table after we eat a meal – automatic.

MOVEMENT	CALORIES BURNT PER DAY	WEIGHT LOSS OVER A YEAR (lb)
Using a bathroom on a different level of your office building	120	9
Getting off public transport a stop early	100	8
Walking a flight of stairs each hour	64	4.5
Getting up every hour and moving for 2 minutes	48	3.5
Getting up to do a chore each ad break when watching TV	36	4.5

Start training

'Walking's good but on its own it's not enough – you have to train.'

It is not uncommon to hear clients describe proudly how they managed to squeeze a 20- or 30-minute walk into their frantic schedule. It may come as a surprise but the human body was built to move a lot, every day. The endless sitting in front of the computer, TV and steering wheel are in fact the exact opposite of the body's design plan, and we have a growing list of lifestyle-related diseases that demonstrate its unhappiness with our sedentary lifestyle. So as we pat ourselves on the back for walking around the block or completing a few minutes on the treadmill, we are really just making up for part of the time we've spent sitting.

While walking will help burn the calories you have ingested over the day and keep your muscles active and burning, to actually lose weight and keep the muscles working at their best, they need to be trained. Training, as opposed to walking, requires your muscles to be stressed, your heart rate to be high and your blood to be pumping. This challenges every cell to burn more fuel and, as a result, improves fitness and cell function. Such training will keep the body at its best rather than simply preventing it from further age-related decline.

But don't be scared – training doesn't mean spending hours inside a hot, sweaty gym. If you're already walking every day, training can simply equate to three or four high-intensity cardio sessions for 20–30 minutes each week: a quick workout on the cross trainer, some interval work on the treadmill and a jog instead of a walk. Focusing on quality rather than quantity when it comes to your training means it won't be such a burden on your already full schedule. You can fit a 20–30-minute workout easily into your lunch break, children's sporting classes or before breakfast. A very simple rule that may help you keep on track when it comes to exercise intensity is that if you are not hot and sweaty at the end of the session, you have not been working hard enough.

Top 10 tips for regular exercise

1   Schedule your training sessions at the start of each week.
2   Prioritise your training sessions.
3   Choose exercise that you enjoy.
4   Don't overcommit to exercise.
5   Don't fall off the wagon entirely if you miss a session.
6   Change your sessions regularly.
7   Move as much as you can every day.
8   Exercise to nurture, not torture, your body.
9   Think quality over quantity when it comes to training.
10 Accept that exercise is something that you will have to do forever.

Learn to interval train

'If you are reading a magazine on the exercise bike, you are not pedalling hard enough.'

If you take a look around any gym floor during peak times, I would estimate that 50 per cent of gym users at most are exercising efficiently. Some are watching TV, others reading books or magazines while on their machine. In most cases, these people could and should be burning a lot more calories.

Once you've reached a good level of fitness, interval training is the best way to train efficiently. This means altering the intensity of training at 1-minute intervals to challenge yourself every workout. For the die-hard treadmill fans, this means increasing the incline; for the bike lovers it means turning up the resistance. If you train outdoors the same principle applies – run in between lampposts or seek out some hills. Anything that changes your heart rate and challenges your body will benefit your weight loss and metabolism long-term.

If you consider that you burn more calories in 20 minutes of solid interval training than you do in 40 minutes of regular cardio training, you can see the benefits from both a time management and energy output perspective. Ideally we need to be burning 80–100 calories per 10 minutes to be able to say that we've had a decent workout.

Time to lift

'Lifting weights or resistance training is the best way to teach your body to burn calories.'

It's one thing to eat less to lose weight, and another to move more, but if you're really going to get control of your weight once and for all, you need to teach your body to burn its food better by building muscle tissue.

Resistance training refers to any type of training that places weighted stress on the muscle, which requires it to build and strengthen its cells. Basically, the more muscle mass you have, the more calories you burn. In addition to that, the more your muscles are worked, the better they become at burning, meaning they become more efficient at burning the food you eat. As most of us like to eat and want to be able to eat as much as we like, teaching your muscles to burn energy better is a powerful thing you can do to improve your metabolic rate.

Like all training regimes, the type of resistance training you do is crucial. Ideally you want to be stressing the muscle, which means increasing the weight you can lift over time. For those who have never done any form of resistance training, starting with light weights will see the body respond well initially. Circuit-style classes that include light hand weights and supported-weights machines tick this box. If you are already fit, more specialised resistance-style programmes may be required.

If you feel that you've been training for some time with no results, or doing the same gym class or personal training session for months with no change to your body shape or size, it's time to check if your training programme is up to scratch.

The best option is to consult a highly experienced personal trainer or exercise physiologist to develop a programme that is exactly right for you. If this isn't an option, make sure that you are increasing the weight you are lifting and/or increasing the number of sets. Generally speaking, women need to do four to five sets of 12–15 repetitions with lighter weights. If you always use supported-weights machines, try swapping to free weights. If you usually train at night, swap to morning sessions or if you always train by yourself, try a boot camp style of training for a change. Remember that the body responds well metabolically to change and challenge. If you are already lifting, you are likely to simply need a change of routine. If you have never lifted, your muscles are waiting for a good workout so get out there.

The body will respond well to even one session a week that has a resistance-training component. For the best results, lifting weights either as part of a programme or as a specific weights session in the gym, two to three times each week, will see maximum benefit in terms of both body composition and metabolic rate.

Check your calories

*'Too many active people are running on empty
and then wonder why they cannot lose weight.'*

One of the most common diet scenarios I see is individuals, particularly
females, training regularly but eating fewer calories than a bedridden
70-year-old female needs. Once you're training at a high level (at least an
hour each day) you cannot ruthlessly cut calories without your metabolic
rate being negatively affected. In fact, the further you reduce your calories,
the less likely it is that you're going to lose weight. Your body will be
fighting to store any extra fat as it is effectively being starved of nutrients.

Once you are training regularly, the lowest caloric intake you should allow
yourself is no fewer than 1500 calories. If you're training for more than an
hour a day, you need to increase this by at least 100–200 calories for every
extra hour of activity you do. This will ensure you don't compromise your
metabolic rate too greatly because the body will have adequate fuel for
the amount of activity it is required to do.

Another option for those training hard and cutting calories without
results is to actually reduce your training. A break from your regular
training schedule while keeping calories relatively low is sometimes all
you need to give your muscles a break and your body a chance to reboot
and get back in touch with its natural hunger and satiety signals.

Caloric checklist for training

- Am I eating at least 1500 calories each day?
- Am I eating 100–200 calories extra per hour of intense activity?
- Am I eating breakfast early?
- Am I moving as well as training?
- Am I checking my heart rate when training?
- Am I being careful to not over-train?

If you're unsure why your weight isn't changing, make sure you're accurately measuring both your caloric intake as well as your caloric output. Often we're simply not aware of the extra calories slipping in, so keep a diet diary for a few days and enter all the food and drink you consume. There are dietary analysis packages available, such as 'calorieking', but often the simple act of writing everything down will reveal where you're going wrong. In terms of caloric output, the best indirect measure is determined by checking your heart rate while training using a heart rate monitor. As a rough guide, aim for your heart rate to be working at 70–80 per cent of its maximum rate. To calculate this, simply subtract your age from 220 and calculate 70–80 per cent of this number. For example, if you are 40 years old, your ideal heart rate for training would be 135–140bpm (beats per minute). Of course, always check this with your doctor prior to starting a new exercise regime. Sometimes regular exercisers simply become used to their regime and are not challenging themselves enough to get the changes in body composition they're looking for.

As a last resort, you can use a very low-calorie plan for a short period but only if you're prepared to also cut back your training. The most common detox programmes will be 1000–1200 calories. At most, try these programmes for just a week or two to give your metabolism a shake up without causing a significant drop in metabolic rate or causing your body to break down muscle tissue for energy.

Unfortunately a healthy diet doesn't always result in fat loss – remember that the balance for fat loss needs to be quite specific, especially when you only have a small amount to lose. Compare the two meal plans on the following pages, for example. Both are very healthy in terms of nutrition, but only the second will result in weight loss.

Typical healthy diet

Breakfast	2 large slices of toast with spread
Midmorning snack	2 peaches, 200g low-fat yoghurt, regular low-fat latte
Lunch	Thai beef stir-fry (no rice)
Pre-dinner snack	Rice crackers, dip, nuts or crackers
Dinner	Chicken stir-fry (no rice)
Dessert	Small bowl of low-fat ice-cream

As you can see, this diet is pretty healthy – the client has even cut carbohydrates at night. But if we analyse the nutrition breakdown:

    2200 calories
    85g fat
    210g total carbohydrate
    = 45% carbs, 20% protein and 35% fat
    = WEIGHT STABLE

While this may look okay, for slow but sustainable fat loss we need to aim for fewer total calories and an improved ratio of carbs, protein and fat.

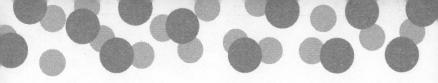

Diet for weight loss

Breakfast	2 slices multigrain toast with poached eggs
Midmorning snack	1 peach, 4 wholegrain crackers with 2 slices low-fat cheese, small low-fat latte
Lunch	Wholegrain bread roll (middle removed) with tuna, thin spread avocado and salad
Midafternoon snack	Cereal bar, rice cakes with low-fat hummus
Dinner	Thai beef salad
Dessert	Low-fat ice-cream on a stick

The nutrition breakdown is:

1600 calories

60g fat

140g total carbohydrate

= 40% carbs, 30% protein and 30% fat

= FAT LOSS

Despite only small differences, this is the better plan for weight loss.

Fuel your body for training

'Sometimes you need carbs to burn more body fat.'

It may surprise you to hear that people who train regularly may struggle to a far greater extent when losing their last bit of weight than those who never train. How can that be?

Regular trainers – those who get up at 5am every weekday and seriously challenge themselves in each session – are adding stress to a body that is also being denied calories. If a muscle is being trained heavily without enough fuel in the form of carbohydrate, metabolic rate will slow down to protect that muscle. If you have not eaten carbs for a prolonged period, such as an overnight fast of 10–12 hours, and the muscles are then pushed to train for another hour in an intense early-morning workout before breakfast, they are unlikely to be operating at their best metabolically to efficiently burn fat. The same can be said for late-afternoon training sessions when no food has been eaten for 4–5 hours, or since lunch. You are likely to feel tired and lethargic (and hence less likely to push yourself in the session), but the muscle will simply not have enough fuel to access fat stores effectively.

So if you're already training for a number of hours each week and know that the intensity is there, it may be time to make sure you're giving your muscles the opportunity to burn fat efficiently. If you train pre-breakfast and have chosen to not eat carbs at dinner the night before, try including a small carbohydrate or protein snack before you train. Just a couple of crackers and a slice of low-fat cheese or half a glass of low-fat milk (or the equivalent of 20g of carbs and 5g of protein) is all you need.

For those who train midmorning, rather than eating a large breakfast early try halving it, that is one slice of toast or half a bowl of cereal to support maximum fat burning during that session. For afternoon exercisers, make sure you include a protein- or carbohydrate-rich snack 1–2 hours before you train. A nut-based snack bar, some thick yoghurt or a protein shake are all good choices.

If you haven't eaten carbs at night for years and expect yourself to train for an hour or more every day, it's time to cut your muscles some slack. Try adding ½–1 cup of cooked carbohydrate to your evening meal. Notice how much better you train with a little fuel on board and how much better you feel as a result.

BEST PRE-TRAINING SNACKS	
MORNING	AFTERNOON
2 crackers + 1 slice low-fat cheese	Nut-based snack bar
1 slice wholegrain toast + peanut butter	Low-fat milk coffee
½ cup milk	150g thick yoghurt
½ low-GI muesli bar	4 crackers + 2 slices low-fat cheese
2 tbsp yoghurt	4 corn thins + peanut butter

your
LIFE

'Ultimately it's your food, your behaviour, your body and your life – how do you want to live it?'

Balancing food and work

'Is your office environment conducive to weight control?'

Michelle was a slim size 10 when she started working at a large law firm. The new job was great. Her boss took her to all the work lunches and the other assistants were always inviting her out for Friday night drinks. After only 3 months, Michelle noticed her skirts were tight and was shocked to discover she had gained 11lb. How had it happened?

Given we spend at least 8 hours a day there, our work environment, whether it be an office, truck or classroom, has a strong influence on the way we eat. The biscuit tin, coffees, celebratory morning teas and vending machines are just some of the temptations we're exposed to. When this extra eating is coupled with sedentary jobs and commutes, it's no surprise that slow, inconspicuous weight gain often results. Of course you can't be a purist and avoid every morning tea, but it's helpful to understand the common food traps at work and ways to avoid them.

Keeping treats out of sight is a good starting point. Put biscuits and chocolates away so they're not staring you in the face. Allocate set times for morning and afternoon tea and don't eat in between. Always keep a supply of filling snacks in the drawer or fridge, so you have healthy choices when hungry. If there seems to be a cake every second day for someone's birthday, wedding or new baby, see if you can organise one day a month for all celebrations to take place.

Be wary of the work lunch. Meals eaten out tend to have double the calories of your standard tuna and salad sandwich. If you find yourself eating out more than once a week, be strict and stick to light salads, soups and grills. Always order extra vegetables or salad and have a light meal that evening to compensate. The food may be delicious but it's likely you'll enjoy delicious meals out on the weekend too.

Being strict with your food intake at work may seem pedantic, but the harsh reality is that we spend up to a third of our lives there and bad habits at work tend to translate into serious weight gain if we're not careful.

WORKPLACE CALORIE TRAPS	
FOOD	CALORIES
200g pack of chocolate	950
Takeaway pasta with pesto	810
Thai rice and meat dish	380
Café-style muffin	310
1 slice of banana bread	240
Large low-fat caramel latte	240
10 jelly beans	110
2 plain sweet biscuits	80

Manage your stress

'Stress is part of busy, modern life, so stress management is crucial if you want to be at your best.'

Do you know anyone who doesn't complain of being stressed at some point? Work pressures, tight schedules and intense interpersonal interactions are common reasons for feeling stressed or overwhelmed. In small doses, stress can be good for us. It gets the blood pumping and improves concentration when experienced in small doses. But chronically high stress levels can impair immune function, mood and wellbeing.

People respond differently to stress. Some become withdrawn and anxious, others compensate with alcohol, drugs or food. For those who use food as comfort, the link between eating and stress is likely to have been formed when they were young. Crying babies are often soothed with food when they may just be looking for touch or attention. The media fuels the link between eating and stress with such terms as 'comfort food' and chocolate biscuit ads during cold winter months.

Research from New York University found a link between stress and eating. The study showed that pre-menopausal women who produce more cortisol (the hormone involved in the body's response to stress) consume more calories and sweet-tasting food when stressed compared to women who produce less cortisol. While not everyone is susceptible to emotional eating, the weight gain for those who are can be significant.

A study comparing normal versus overweight women's emotional responses to stress found that the more a woman weighed, the more likely she was to eat in response to negative moods and situations.

While a sugar hit can make us feel momentarily better, the key to managing stress-based eating is learning to manage the stressor itself. This means learning to develop clear strategies for identifying, managing and reducing the stress in our lives. To break the link between stress and eating, put some time between the stressful event and eating. Go for a walk, a drive or call a friend. Don't give yourself permission to eat simply because you are stressed – stress is a normal part of life and we need to manage it. If you find that putting something in your mouth does soothe you somewhat, try munching on a carrot, gum or even a lollipop to create the physical stimulation without a calorie overload.

Top 10 stress-less techniques

1   Move your body each day.
2   Express gratitude for something that is great in your life.
3   Take time out to chat to someone close to you each day.
4   Grow something.
5   Cut your TV viewing time by half.
6   Smile at one new person each day.
7   Phone a close friend.
8   Have a good belly laugh.
9   Do one nice thing for yourself each day.
10 Do something nice for someone else.

Travel smart

'Never let yourself become a victim of your environment.'

When busy professionals come in for an appointment, it is rarely a lack of knowledge preventing them from reaching their health and fitness goals. Rather it is a busy lifestyle and not paying enough attention to planning that sees them becoming a victim of their environment. Regular business trips, lunches, air travel and hotel stays coupled with a lack of planning and eating what is available as opposed to what they should be eating. Over time this equates to weight gain rather than weight loss.

If you consider that the standard snack served on domestic flights contains more than 350 calories, or a quarter of a female's daily calorie requirement, and up to 60g of carbohydrate, or the equivalent of 4 slices of bread, it is easy to see where things can go off track so easily.

The way you can ensure that you keep on track with your diet and exercise regime, even if you travel regularly, is by keeping your food routine as stable as possible no matter where you're going. Always travel with protein-rich snacks and fruit, and get into the habit of saying no when other food is served, knowing it is unlikely to be of the quality you require. Make a concerted effort to get out of the hotel to a local supermarket to keep your breakfast foods and snacks on hand, and remember that if you're paying for hotel service, staff will often be more than happy to prepare the specific salads, wraps and even snacks you request, even if you have to pay a little extra for them.

When it comes to work lunches, if they are pre-orders, put in a special dietary request in advance to ensure you will be served enough protein and salad or grab a sandwich or sushi in the morning to take with you. Eating out is no excuse. No matter which restaurant or food outlet you go to, there will be good choices. Base your meals around lean proteins and always order extra sides of vegetables or salad. You don't have to be a food purist if you're dining at a top restaurant as a one-off, but if you travel regularly you'll need to keep your dietary regime on track if you really want to lose or even just control your weight.

Another thing to remember is that for many of us, travelling actually provides an opportunity to move more. All of a sudden typical time drainers – including commuting, children and partners, or no easy access to a gym – are eliminated, making it far easier to find 30 minutes to get to the hotel gym or go for a quick walk before breakfast. Look to your travel time as an opportunity to move more, not less.

Get a daily timetable

'No time is a poor excuse – we all have 24 hours in a day. How do you use yours?'

Every single person I know is busy. How many people do you know who regularly say, 'I have a spare hour, what can I do with it?' Long working hours, long commutes, bulging social diaries all contribute to extremely full schedules and a constant lack of time to do the things that we really want to. In saying that, we all have 24 hours a day. Some of us manage to do a lot with that time and others far less, which means we need to be better with our time management if we are to fit regular exercise and healthy eating into our day.

An easy way to work out how you could become more efficient and free up some time for a healthy lifestyle is to work out where you currently spend your time and more importantly, where you waste it. Simply make a template of your entire 24 hours, and fill in the spaces over a week. The most common areas people waste time are watching mindless TV and the advertisements that go with it, commuting, getting out of bed late and surfing the internet. While there is nothing wrong with watching a little TV or relaxing, doing it out of habit and fatigue as opposed to interest is where we waste time.

Once you are aware of where your time goes, you can start to develop strategies to become more efficient. Taping shows you like and watching them without the advertisements, trying to drive outside peak times, getting up early and fitting in some exercise – all of these are examples of ways that busy people get things done in their world.

To really be in control of your weight and your body, you need to have a very clear idea of what you need to do each day to support your health goals, and how you are going to fit these things into your schedule. Once you are aware of these steps, documenting them and practising them until they become a daily habit will be the act that converts your health desires into your health outcomes.

So this week, as you sit at your computer with your morning coffee, start to make a list of all the things you need to do each day to make sure you eat well and exercise. Then factor all the items into your weekly timetable. Print it out and stick it up by your computer. A regular glance at it will remind you that you need to make yourself a cup of green tea, or walk upstairs to the bathroom to get your step number up. Remember, it's the little things that add up and lead to positive long-term health outcomes.

Sacred Sunday

'Sunday is the day to get ready for the week ahead
so that come Monday you hit the ground running.'

Sundays are often just as busy as every other day of the week with social functions and even work taking over this traditional day of rest. This usually means we fall into bed late on Sunday night, even more exhausted than we were on Friday, dreading the week ahead. If this sounds familiar, it's time to instate Sacred Sundays.

Sacred Sunday means setting aside one day every week when nothing is planned, so you can prepare for a healthy week ahead. You need to greet each Monday with a week's supply of healthy food so you start the week on the right foot. Sacred Sunday gives you time to shop for the food you need to eat well, time to prepare a couple of meals so you have some back-up options for those late nights home, and time to move your body. A good night's sleep on Sunday also makes you less likely to skip the all-important Monday workout.

Part of Sacred Sunday is also to set goals for the week, so as you relax in bed or in front of the TV, make a note of three to five things you hope to achieve in the week ahead. Small but steady and regular progress on our goals brings us closer to achieving them.

You have the power to manage your weight

*'You now have the tools you need to manage your weight –
the question is, will you choose to use them?'*

As we approach the end of this book, you will have some new diet and
lifestyle tricks that you've started to implement and that you will be able
to maintain for many years to come. I also hope you come away feeling
motivated and positive as you finally move forward with your health goals.

Although some of these new weight-loss tricks are exciting, deep down
we all know how to look after our bodies. We need to eat less and move
more. We know that we need to cut back at times, and when we need to
take our training or food choices to a new level. If we are truly honest with
ourselves, we know what holds us back.

As is the case with any behavioural change process, you will make the
changes at the exact time that things are right for you to do so. Listening
and trusting yourself is often the step we need to take to cement things.
So from today, know that you now have the knowledge, the tools and the
mental strength you need to manage your weight. Once you cement this
belief, you can only move forward.

Victim no more

'I can never lose weight, it's not fair.'

The sooner you stop playing the weight-loss victim, the sooner you'll gain control of your weight, health and fitness. The same can be said for life – some of us are always the victim. We don't have enough money, time, hate our job, have an awful boyfriend holding us back, and the list goes on.

So, are you a victim of your own life? Do you constantly complain but do nothing to change your circumstance? Do you spend time with people who never tend to move forward? Do you bring energy to others or do you drain it?

Many of us earn a victim mentality when small via parents or early school experiences, but it's never too late to identify and make positive changes to reverse it.

When I first meet a new client in a weight-loss consultation, I can tell almost immediately if they are going to succeed with their weight-loss goals. Individuals who are ready to change have a very different attitude to those who are there hoping that I will pull out my magical weight-loss wand and hit them on the head with it. Those who succeed are looking for the opportunity to get their weight under control, are open to new ideas and draw on their personal resources to be able to make the often simple life changes they need to take control.

The truth be known, we are all incredibly lucky – lucky to have the bodies we complain about, lucky to have easy access to good-quality food, lucky to have all the opportunities we easily take for granted. It's time to embrace that luck and think about ways we can make the most of it. To be grateful for the body we've been given, nurture it with good food and keep it healthy with plenty of movement. To accept that life in general is challenging but rewarding if we actively seek to improve it rather than wallow and complain.

There is no easy way out when it comes to weight control. The majority of us need to eat well most of the time and move regularly. It's as simple or complex as you choose to make it.

CHANGE YOUR MINDSET	
VICTIM RESPONSE	OPPORTUNIST RESPONSE
I wish I could eat what I want.	Few people can really eat what they want.
I can never lose weight.	Everyone can lose weight if they do it the right way for them.
I gain weight no matter what I eat.	You will only gain weight if you are eating too many calories.
Weight loss is so hard.	Everything is hard when you first start.
Weight loss should be easy.	The benefits of weight loss are too huge to miss out on.

No more excuses

'Excuses – some of us make them, others take responsibility and refuse to bow down to them.'

Have you ever wondered why some people reach their goals and stay on track no matter what, and others always have an excuse why they haven't done what they said they would do? If you are really committed to getting your weight under control for good, you have to get rid of your excuses. No more excuses as to why you missed your workout. No more excuses as to why you ate rubbish for lunch. Why you skipped your walk. Why you did not have the foods at work you need to eat well.

Successful people do not make excuses. They do what they need to do to make sure things happen. They take charge and schedule training sessions they know they will get to. They prepare their food no matter where they are in the world. They work as hard as they need to get things done. And if and when they do occasionally go off track, they get right back on it.

Are you an excuse maker? Do you regularly change your schedule so that eating well and exercising take a back seat? Do you eat rubbish when you could have eaten better with a little extra effort and focus? One of the most common reasons we make excuses for not doing what we said we would is that the goals we have set are not in line with our own values and personal likes. We commit to a gym membership even though we hate the gym or try to follow a diet that we loathe. It's crucial to develop an eating plan and exercise regime that's realistic and right for you.

The next thing you can do to move away from the excuse mindset is to be aware of the times you are making excuses. When you feel an excuse coming on, rather than take the easy option, look for other alternatives to ensure you keep your lifestyle goals on track.

Once you eliminate the option for excuses, all of a sudden you are free from psychological limitations and can move forward with your weight loss. Remember that many of our behaviours are habits – habits that have become deeply entrenched after years of practice. If you have always come up with excuses that prevent you from reaching your weight-loss goals, they will keep popping up until you eradicate them. Don't give yourself a choice – just commit.

Rejecting laziness

'Are you tired? Overworked? Or are you just lazy?'

It's easy to be lazy living in a society where food is abundant and living standards are high. We leave garages and drive to offices with undercover parking. We have people to deliver our shopping, calculate our tax and take care of our dry cleaning, but when health or fitness professionals suggest moving our bodies more, we take the advice begrudgingly.

Living in a blessed world is sadly a large part of the reason so many of us are fat and unfit. We're quick to make excuses for not preparing our own food or to explain why we missed a gym session. We are quick to blame our laziness on fatigue or a low mood but the truth is to make long-term lifestyle changes that support weight control, we need to be strict, identify our lazy behaviour and put a stop to it.

Do you routinely switch off the morning alarm or cancel training sessions? Do you often find yourself eating fast food because you're too lazy to spend an extra 10 minutes preparing a more nutritious dinner? Do you grab quick high-fat snacks on the run because you are too lazy to go to the supermarket and stock up on more nutritious snack food options? We are all time poor and have a lot going on but some people manage to get things done and keep their diet on track, and some don't. Which do you want to be?

See only solutions

'I don't want to hear what went badly,
I only want to hear what went well.'

When clients return for a weight-loss review after their first appointment, it's common for them to spend the first few minutes outlining all the things they've done wrong or not completed. The scary thing is that starting any dialogue with such a negative mindset has been proven to narrow our brain's ability to identify opportunities and strategies to move forward. We talk ourselves into failure.

It is imperative when committing to long-term behavioural change and sustainable weight loss that we remain solution-focused at all times – that is, looking only for answers, not problems. Seeking ways to move forward rather than dwelling on what has not come together, seeking answers to apparent problems rather than complaining, being on the constant look out for new opportunities, for good to come from apparent bad, being positive, all the time.

It's very easy to fall into old thought patterns and habits when it comes to weight loss; 'Weight loss is so hard', 'I can never lose weight', 'Diets never work for me', or 'I don't have time for exercise'. Each of these declarations is negative in both tone and direction. A simple shift towards the positive, 'This time I will lose weight for good', 'This time I will lose weight no matter what', 'I will find the right dietary balance for me', 'I will find time to exercise every day', is all you need to start looking for opportunities to control your weight as opposed to reasons not to.

If you think about it, the role of a health professional in the weight-loss process is simply to help brainstorm ideas that will help you progress. To think about dietary options and new foods to try that will help achieve the ideal dietary balance, to brainstorm new exercise options, to support, problem solve and move you forward. And you too can do this simply by always remaining solution-focused on your weight-loss journey. Waste no time dwelling on problems that arise – instead view them as a way to take the next step and move forward. Know that there is always an answer and that road humps are simply part of any change and new process.

Once you adopt a solution-only approach you will be surprised how much easier life becomes. Precious time and energy is no longer wasted on things we cannot control, but channelled into making our goals achieveable.

Commit to self-care

'Be your best for you, and then for those around you.'

Men are much better at it than women, and mothers are the worst of all. Our weight, mood and health suffer when we don't do it, but it can be a challenging habit to build and maintain – self-care. Although it seems like a basic biological function, much time is spent in diet consultations helping people learn the importance of self-care – the daily need to keep body, mood and health in good shape so we can be at our best.

The mistake many of us make is not prioritising our own needs, instead giving everything to others before we consider caring for ourselves. This leaves us tired, grumpy, overweight and resentful while teaching others that this is okay, so friends and family continue to expect it. If you know you need to work on your self-care, here are some starting ideas:

1 Aim for at least one fun social event each week.
2 Aim to do one nice thing for yourself each week.
3 Aim for some alone time with your partner at least once a month.
4 Schedule at least three exercise sessions each week.
5 Plan at least one break or holiday to look forward to each year.

Once you create these breaks in your life, you'll be surprised how much better you feel, and how much more energy you have to make the effort to eat well and move your body.

Commit to a steely mindset

'Allow nothing to distract you from your health and lifestyle goals.'

Life is full of distractions – situations, people and opportunities that cross our path on an hourly, daily, yearly basis. We can either choose to engage with them or continue along our self-directed path. Some people are exceptionally good at ignoring distractions, quickly determining whether they are in line with their big-picture plan. Others spend their lives being distracted by other people or life in general and never really achieve any of their goals. These people often feel unsatisfied and unfulfilled, wondering where on earth the time went, and why they're in exactly the same place they were 5 years ago.

The same can be said for those people who manage to stay on track with their weight-loss goals and those who don't. People who stay on track don't skip their walk or workout for a shopping trip. They say no to an extra glass of wine or dessert because they know what they need to do to stay healthy and feel good.

Developing a steely mindset when it comes to your food and training regimes will take time, especially if it's a new thing for you. First of all it will require you to clearly define your goals. Next you need to identify distracters – the people, events, media and other stimuli that take you off track, physically or mentally – and develop strategies to ignore them.

Learn to avoid and ignore the countless hours of mindless chatter with people who will not be a part of your life long-term, to avoid and ignore the constant media stream in which we waste so much time and energy, to avoid and ignore people in our world who drain our energy and leave us less inclined to go about achieving our goals.

At times this may mean missing social engagements we didn't want to go to anyway, or that we have no idea what's happening on the latest TV show, but it will also mean we have more time to look after ourselves. And the more we nurture and look after ourselves, the better the position we find ourselves in to manage our weight long-term.

Identifying distracters

- Will I have any regrets if I don't participate in this event?
- Will this person be in my life in 1, 5 or 10 years?
- What could I achieve if I don't do this?
- What is the most important thing I can do with my time right now?
- In my life, which people, events and activities bring me the most pleasure?
- What's the worst thing that can happen if I don't do this?

Cement your new habits

'It takes 3 days to become aware of a new habit and up to 3 months before an old habit is replaced, so be patient.'

Habits – the things we do day in, day out without thinking – are crucial when it comes to developing sustainable diet and exercise changes. Developing a new habit is all very well but cementing it to become a long-term regular part of your day is something else. Now you have come this far, here are the key habits that we know are linked to weight control long-term and that you need to cement if you are to improve your food, your body and your life, for good.

1. ALWAYS EAT BREAKFAST
People who eat a substantial breakfast lose more weight than those who have a small breakfast. Choose eggs or baked beans on wholegrain bread, natural muesli with fruit and yoghurt or a liquid meal drink and notice how much more satisfied you feel throughout the morning.

2. EAT 3 CUPS OF VEGETABLES AND TWO FRUITS EACH DAY
Having half your plate filled with vegetables or salad at lunch and dinner helps to tick this box, as does adding fruit to your breakfast and vegetable for a snack on the way home from work.

3. TAKE TIME TO SHOP EACH WEEK

If the food is not in the house, how can you eat well? Schedule in time to shop each week and use online options if you hate spending time in a busy supermarket.

4. WALK 10,000 STEPS A DAY

Remember this is on top of your regular exercise routine. A pedometer is extremely useful in providing feedback on how many steps you are racking up every day.

5. SIT DOWN AT THE TABLE TO EAT

You will eat more slowly and often eat less food as a result. Remember eating is supposed to be an enjoyable and social experience so take time out to do it properly.

6. ALWAYS CARRY A HEALTHY SNACK

Most of us know what the good food choices are – the problem arises when we get hungry and don't have nutritious food options with us and end up eating high-fat food on the run. Great options to keep handy include cereal or protein snack bars, hard fruit (such as an apple) or a few crackers so you're never caught off guard.

7. DRINK GREEN TEA AFTER MEALS

Not only is green tea exceptionally high in antioxidants, it can also help increase metabolic rate and curb sugar cravings.

8. ALWAYS CARRY A WATER BOTTLE

Once again, if it's in front of you, you will drink it. Aim for at least two bottles of water each day as a replacement for juice, cordial or soft drinks.

9. CHOOSE WHOLEGRAIN, LOW-GI BREAD AND CEREALS

Aim for the best-quality bread, crackers and breakfast cereal as these are foods we eat every day. Choose low-GI, wholegrain pastas, cereals and breads that are portion-controlled such as small slices of multigrain bread and measured portions of breakfast cereal, rice and pasta.

10. EAT CARBS AND PROTEIN FOR OPTIMAL SATIETY

Low-GI carbohydrates provide sustainable energy, while protein offers key nutrients and helps to keep us full. Some examples are eggs on multigrain toast, yogurt and fruit, crackers and cheese or wholegrain bread with tuna, chicken or salmon.

Maintain your motivation

'You can have anything if you want it enough.'

Motivation is a complex and changeable state. For many, it's innate when it comes to health and fitness. For others, a health scare or realisation that they're four sizes bigger than they should be provides the kick needed to turn their lives around. Then there are those who just never get it. They try one health and fitness craze after the other, never cementing a pattern of living that works for them and gives their bodies a better chance.

If you have reached this point in the book, it's safe to say that you're motivated and keen to stay that way. To achieve your goals, you'll need strategies to maintain this motivation by regularly reminding yourself why you've committed to important diet and exercise changes long-term. Some simple questions that may help you to clarify your reasons for wanting to stay fit and healthy include:

- What are the benefits of keeping my body fit and healthy?
- How would my life be better if I felt better about my body?
- Am I a healthy role model for my children?
- Can I physically do all the things I would like to?
- If I was fit, healthy and happy what would I be eating and what training would I be doing each day?
- If I knew I could help keep my body disease-free by eating well and exercising, would I be more inclined to move more and eat less?

- Who are the people in my life who would support me living like this?
- What changes can I make to my lifestyle today that will help move me closer to my goal of living well and feeling good?

Having clear answers to these questions reminds you of the bigger reasons for wanting to get in shape and stay there. Keep these answers on hand and refer back to them if you find yourself going off track. A simple and proven technique to maintain motivation for healthy living is to make a visual reminder of these questions and answers and place them somewhere where you will see them every day. When we repeatedly remind ourselves of the reasons why we make simple daily decisions, it helps reinforce the key behaviours and habits we need to stay on track. Keep a copy of these mantras at work, in the car or in your mobile so you can take control and pull yourself back in line.

For behavioural change to be sustained long-term, the reason for wanting it in the first place needs to come from within. It cannot be based on wanting to look good for a wedding or to fit into a certain dress – the motivation has to become so entrenched that you can no longer imagine life without it. As you embrace this new approach to weight loss and start to take control of your health, give yourself 3 months to cement your new habits. Then the longer you maintain these habits after that 3-month period, the harder they will be to break.

Embrace your true self

'Be kind to yourself.'

Time after time, seasoned dieters attend a new diet appointment or read another magazine and mentally commit to the latest diet or training programme. Yet after a day, week or month, the regime falls apart and they're back to where they started, feeling worse about themselves than ever before. It's an exhausting, boring, predictable cycle that achieves nothing.

The most important step you can take towards ending this vicious cycle is to be kind to yourself. Consider what you really need – from your relationships, work, social life and diet and exercise regime. Figuring this out has to come from approaching self-care positively, not from a position of frustration where you beat yourself up for being fat and lazy. The negative mindset instantly talks you into failure and gives you excuses to revert to old habits. So don't punish yourself – give yourself a break.

Once you start being kind to yourself and nourishing your mind and body with exercise and the right amount of good-quality food, you'll be in the perfect position to determine the best way forward in looking after yourself for life. You will move beyond the diet and exercise baggage that has literally weighed you down for too long and enjoy the lifestyle that makes you feel good. You are free to enjoy what life has waiting for you – so get on with it, the time is now.

Acknowledgements

This book would not have been possible without the ongoing love and support of many. Thank you to Lisa Wilkinson, a mentor whose wise words gave me the inspiration and confidence to bring these ideas together. To Helen Wellings, who provided professional guidance and moral support throughout the entire process.

To Pippa from Curtis Brown, who believed in this project from the beginning, as did my amazing publishers from Hardie Grant – Fran Berry, Paul McNally and Julie Pinkham, who made this process so enjoyable. A special thanks to my beautiful editor Bel Monypenny, who not only did a magnificent job but was an absolute pleasure to work with. To Jenny Macmillan and Rosalind McClintock – you too have been dreams to work with.

Next, to those whose support and patience I will be forever grateful. To Anna Louise Bouvier, Sharron Flahive, Katie Marks, Alex 'Possy' Portelli, Kerryn 'Bartrop' Chisholm and the 'family', Janene Theol, my darling B, Georgie, Pete, and the world's best trainer Dave Driscoll. To Emma, Kat and Pepps – you make my workdays so much more enjoyable. I look forward to more baking, laughs, poetry and life lessons.

And finally, but most importantly, to my parents Jeff and Leah. This book would never have been completed without you. I love you with all my heart.

Published in 2011 by Hardie Grant Books

Hardie Grant Books (UK)
Dudley House, North Suite
34–35 Southampton Street
London WC2E 7HF
www.hardiegrant.co.uk

Hardie Grant Books (Australia)
85 High Street
Prahran, Victoria 3181
www.hardiegrant.com.au

Cataloguing-in-Publication data is available from the British Library.
Losing the Last 10lb: Simple steps to get the body you want now

ISBN 978 1 74270 048 9

Cover design by Trisha Garner
Text design and typesetting by Jacqueline Richards
Printed and bound in the UK by CPI Cox & Wyman, Reading, RG1 8EX

Other titles by Hardie Grant Books

OMG! I Can Eat That?

By Jane Kennedy

PUBLICATION DATE January 2011
PRICE £14.99 Paperback

Like most of us, Jane Kennedy can't eat anything she wants because she gets FAT. After having five children in six years and trying every fad diet known to man, Jane decided to take matters into her own hands. A lifetime love of cooking, teamed with a refusal to give up the flavours of her favourite meals, led Jane to develop her own dishes that are delicious but also good for you.

In *OMG! I can eat that?*, Jane shares some of her favourite indulgent recipes, just without all the unwanted fat. These recipes aren't your typical 'diet' recipes, with delicious meals such as Beef Bourguignon, Boombah-free Burgers, and even sweet treats like Rhubarb and Strawberry Crumble, you'll forget you're even eating food minus the boombah!

ISBN 9781740669924

Fabulous Food, Minus the Boombah

by Jane Kennedy

PUBLICATION DATE June 2011
PRICE £14.99 Paperback

In Fabulous food, minus the boombah, Jane shares the recipes that
allowed her to lose weight and feel fantastic: meals for every
day in the home, for entertaining, for nights when you can't be bothered
cooking and just really want takeaway, and even some pretty deceptively
delicious desserts.

Jane Kennedy: Fabulous Food Minus the Boombah is your new way of
cooking – packed full of flavour but minus the boombah!

ISBN 9781740668088

Feel Good Food
By Tony Chiodo

PUBLICATION DATE February 2011
PRICE £16.99 Paperback

Food has the potential not only to taste good and be good for you,
but to make you feel good too. And with Tony Chiodo's recipes
you'll be eating well and feeling better than ever before.

Try Baby Leek and Asparagus Salad with Miso Dressing, Seared
Tuna with Sticky Shitake Sauce, or indulge in Carrot, Cardamon
and Coconut Cake

The perfect book for anyone who wants to eat well and feel great,
Feel Good Food will help anyone with an interest in healthy eating
become a confident wholefood masterchef.

ISBN 9781740668873